Cassandra —

I loved
meeting
You!

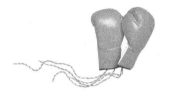

I Am the One

How a Lunge Across the Room
Launched a Woman's Fierce
Fight Against Cancer!

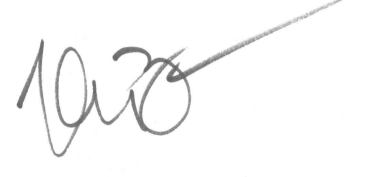

Viki Zarkin

I AM THE ONE
Copyright ©2021 By Viki Zarkin

Published by:
Viki Zarkin Enterprises, LLC
IAmTheOne.com
IAmTheOne.Viki@gmail.com

ISBN: 978-1-7378729-0-0 (hardcover)
ISBN: 978-1-7378729-1-7 (ebook)

What would you do if you were
told to go home and die?
One woman who decided a rare and deadly cancer
wouldn't stop her from raising her children ...

Contents

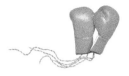

Foreword

Viki Zarkin was 44 in 2010 when she understood the diagnosis a woman or man should ever have to receive from a doctor: "It was simple: There was nothing they could do for me. I had stage 4 metastatic cancer. He was very sorry. But I should go home and get my affairs in order."

What she replied describes the new invincible Viki born that day.

"I will do ANYTHING. Pain, needles, medicine, I don't care how much pain you cause me. I'm a MOM! I want to raise my children. Don't you understand? I'm GOING TO BE THE ONE. I'm going to MAKE it!"

For the past eleven years, that is exactly how Viki Zarkin has led her life: insisting she is THE ONE who will make it and continuing against all odds to be just that. Anyone who knows Viki Zarkin knows that the most important word in her life is FAMILY. Thus, when Viki was faced with the toughest struggle of her life, she knew she would fight with every ounce of her being, not for herself, but for her family. "Surrender" was no more a part of her vocabulary than "farewell" to her family. So, she did what anyone who knew and loved Viki would expect: Fight like hell to overcome this abominable cancer and stay alive.

And now, eleven years after the initial diagnosis, as a top, highly sought-after inspirational speaker who was showcased on the famous Reuters Billboard in Times Square, Viki is still standing, her body understandably weakened by years of invasive chemotherapy, radical surgeries, and experimental radiation. But that doesn't matter. She is still a mother, a wife, a daughter, a sister, a cousin, a niece, and a friend, armed with the strongest weapon on the face of the earth: the deep and passionate love of her family. And what an army this is.

Be prepared for a heart-rending story of pain and triumph, of fear and of courage, and of joy and sorrow... with no tiny detail aspect omitted. What is most exceptional about this story is its ability to grab its readers from its first word and hold them in its thrust until the final sentence has been written. Of course, Viki tells it all, every minute bit, while never losing for one second her indomitable sense of humor. You cannot help but laugh far more than you might cry with this story. But, most of all, you cannot help but adore this woman as much as all her loved ones do. This is not a story of anger and suffering. It is a beautifully written story of love and courage and of hope and gratitude from an extraordinary woman who manages to make every reader feel like a member of her treasured family.

Thanks to I AM THE ONE, no one who faces a dire diagnosis needs ever to feel alone, for Viki details her own struggle in vivid and touching stories; her unique 'Vikiness" evident in her every word. Her ability to find her own voice to tell her difficult story with humor rather than "Why me?" cannot be underestimated. Viki would far rather have her reader laugh with her than in any way grieve for her. For pity has no place in this woman's life. Her hopeful yet honest words pull her readers into her home, her heart, and her story, and those are good places to be.

By, Phyllis Karis New York Times Best Seller For *Brutal: The Untold Story Of My Life Inside Whitey Bulger's Irish Mob*

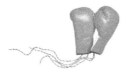

Prologue

They tell me I'm the only one like me alive. Weird ... me? I feel kinda like a circus act. I guess you're going to want to know what all this means. I'm game to try, but if you figure anything out along the way, could you clue me in? Anyway, this is one of those long stories, so you might want to get a snack.

So, here it is in the simplest terms: I have one of those aggressive types of cancers, the kind that really grabs hold and doesn't let go—the kind of cancer that you are going to die from whether it's from the disease or from complications from the treatments. It's like a Catch-22 deal: You die from cancer, or you die painfully from organ failure. Either way, the palm reader will tell you that you don't have a long lifeline, understood? I suppose I should back up here and explain, but I'm not always great at that, so buckle up and hold on tight. I'll say I'm sorry in advance.

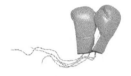

The Mammogram

I always got my mammograms yearly. I was pretty good about that and in 2010 at age forty- four, I did not differ from this routine. In truth, I had a few health problems that year, so I was about six months behind. When I was finally having my mammogram procedure in my hometown of Harrisburg, PA, I wasn't the least bit concerned when the radiologist requested more pictures. After all, my breasts have always been cystic, so this sequence of events was typical for me. Even when he asked me to wait for an ultrasound, I wasn't alarmed. As usual, nothing went quickly and smoothly with my breasts. It was never just in and out. It was always something. At least that's how it had always seemed to me.

It began twenty years earlier when at age twenty-three, I had a result that led to surgery to remove a lump that turned out to be benign. That fun procedure took birth control pills off the table for me and introduced an annual trip to the radiologist. To say I was over the whole annoying breast situation and the typical ensuing drama was putting it mildly. It was always a "suspected this and a false that," so by this time, it pretty much went in one ear and out the other. So, when I finally went home, I didn't think much about the test. What I was thinking about was the horrible flu that had suddenly hit me and was now making me feel like crap.

On December 19, 2010, as I was lying in my flu-induced misery and wondering if I would ever feel better again, the phone rang. The words I heard on the other end would change my life forever.

"Viki, you have cancer," my internist, Dr. G., was telling me in a flat and simple sentence. Nauseated and dizzy from the flu and barely able to stop puking even to answer the phone, I could not initially absorb the meaning of those four words. When my head became a bit clearer, my thoughts centered on what I knew about breast cancer. I mean, I knew breast cancer was relatively common for women in my age group. Plus, wasn't it totally curable? So, I had nothing to worry about, right? I, of all people, should know that. That was why I'd been getting a yearly mammogram for twenty years. My breast cancer could not be far advanced. Everything should be fine. However, I did realize it was gonna be a pain in the ass at the very least, for sure, and scary, too. Let's be real. Somewhere deep inside where you're totally pretending to yourself that you will be fine, you're still getting shit scared. But Remember I told myself over and over, "It's curable, so breathe."

So my journey began. It was not an easy beginning when I talked to Dr. G. While he did recommend some local doctors, he also explained that he was very worried and highly recommended I consider connecting with doctors at Johns Hopkins. When I sent all my x-rays off to Hopkins, as well as to the local oncologists, I figured I was in for a long wait. After all, it was the blessed winter holiday season—Christmas, New Year's, everyone's favorite time of year, everyone's favorite vacation time ... and everyone's favorite time to be out of the office until the beginning of the new year. Needless to say, when I received a call from a doctor from Johns Hopkins a mere two days after I sent in the x-rays, well before I heard a word from any local doctors, I thought I was going to throw up or shit my pants, whichever was more convenient at the moment. After all, I was speaking on the phone to the doctor at the time, so just one hole at a time, please, for God sakes. The words urging me to come in for a biopsy right away, immediately after the holidays, pretty much leveled me. BAM, there it was! Shit, now I know I'm in trouble because let's face it, Hopkins doesn't just call—especially that fast—if it's going to be a walk in the park. They saw something bad, and I'm Fucked. Not only am I Fucked but now I must wait until after the holidays, until January fifth to find out what the hell is going on. Are you kidding me!? Why didn't you just call me on the fourth to come in the next day. Seriously. Making me wait till after the holidays—a WHOLE WEEK—was beyond cruel. I was in Doom Time Countdown!

Well, guess what, everybody? Doom Time is way better than reality if you can believe that. Doom Time was ten times better than REALITY TIME, which turned out to be way, way, way worse.

Having survived the week of not knowing, I was now in the even more mentally exhausting world of figuring it out—a world of more tests and more not knowing. This new world involved a full month of daily two-hour drives from Harrisburg to Baltimore for more tests and the two-hour drive back home, repeated for a full thirty days of agony.

From this hideous time, a couple of memories about a couple of particular people stick out the most. They may seem kind of out of place here, but that's the way memory goes. You see, I'm a private person, so until I could get a full diagnosis and my bearings, these two dear local friends were the only people outside my immediate family who knew what was going on. One of the hardest things was that my strong brave bestie had recently suffered a great personal loss due to the same disease that was now mine. I hurt when she hurt and was invested in her loss. Because I loved her, I didn't want to be the face of any pain that I may inadvertently cause her. She has such a big heart, and I knew I would set aside my feelings for hers because she too was a warrior. It was a moment I will always remember in my head and heart. In fact, she'd be surprised to know it's a burden and hurt I still carry with me today. She has been such a bright light through my whole process, and I will always be grateful for her strength, open heart, love, and courage. I could not have survived without her.

My other memory of that time is of a tiny bit of comic relief in an otherwise terrifying situation. The second loving friend who knew what was going on would try to help me all the time with his own "personal touch." When I was scared and didn't know the doctors at Hopkins, he did all the research for me, letting me know all the details about all my doctors, so I could be more relaxed when I met them. But sometimes his personal touch could be really, really clumsy. Before my very first visit to meet a doctor at Hopkins when I was totally lost with worry and fear from all the waiting, my sweet, sweet friend informed me that Dr. E., a doctor with a clearly Jewish last name was not Jewish at all but rather Black and Catholic. I was deeply grateful for all the research he had given me and felt prepared to meet this physician.

Understand, I couldn't have given two hoots what color the guy was; I just wanted to be prepared in every possible way, I guess. It was weirdly comforting to have something of an image of the doctor who would tell me my fate. So, while my husband, my mother, and I sat nervously in the waiting room, we noticed a board with the doctors' photos next to their names. That's when we all saw it: a very large photo of the doctor we're about to see. Yep, you guessed it; he was clearly White—a very White, likely Jewish man just as his name had suggested in the first place. "Hey, friend of mine, who taught you your research skills?! I mean how hard could it have been when the website had the same photograph?!" We laughed at my well-intentioned friend's mistake, releasing some of the pent-up tension. This sweet friend always knows how to lighten the mood even if by accident. He's still the best of the best ... and still tries to take care of me with his clunky personal touch. He has bought every single cancer cookbook available from which he makes the very worst lumpy muffins I have ever tasted in my life. But they are dripping with love, and I will always love him for those god-awful muffins, his horrible advice, and his unwavering love for me.

(Back to the story now.)

The daily back and forth for testing at Hopkins exhausted me. On the drive there, I would think, *okay, today is the day I am finally going to know more, maybe a stage for my cancer.*

Instead, they would say, "Come back tomorrow for this test."

Now let me interrupt myself yet again just to give you a fuller picture. While Mom, Jere, and I were endlessly driving back and forth for the month of January, getting test after test with more and more bad news piling on each day, we would come home to two small children who needed their mother and father. Taking care of them required lots of attention. They had no idea what was going on. After all, what would be the point of telling them when I didn't have a whole story yet. If I hadn't made any sense of it myself, I wasn't in any position to tell my young children what was happening. They were so sweet and impressionable. My goodness, our son Dell was eleven and in fifth grade, our daughter Isabella was eight and in second grade. They wanted to play when we got home, and Dell needed help with homework. These things were important! Little people don't care that you're tired or scared or had a bad day. They wanted their booboos kissed and stories read and read over again, and "Mommy, don't skip the good parts," and "Will you sing to me all the songs at night and rub my back?" Kids need nurturing, and I'm always a mom first. So, you dig deep and suck it up and play and give the bath time and are grateful for it because those little people count on you and hell if you are ever going to let them down!

Finally, after what seemed to be the millionth test, Dr. E. wanted me to do one additional test. He had been very thorough throughout this whole process, and we had gotten quite close. His daughter was becoming a bat-mitzvah in a year, and my Dell was to be a bar-mitzvah in two years, so we had our children in common. It became something for us to talk about. We later found that his daughter played tennis, Dell played soccer, and so on. I liked and trusted him.

That day when he suggested a new test, he had a hunch I knew that this was going to hurt, but I was still game. He explained I was going to need to hold still because the needle could puncture my lung if I moved. Oh, shit! This didn't sound so great. YIKES! And, oh, by the way, he said, "I can't get you numb because I'm going so deep it's not possible." Oh, double shit!! This really doesn't sound good. Now I'm starting to get nervous. I'm thinking my mom and Jere have no idea what's going on here. Better get the smelling salts, just in case. Okay, so I gear up. I am pretty tough, so I'm ready, and he goes for it. Holy shit, it was pain I have never felt before. And I birthed two children. I don't think I have felt pain quite like that since. And I've been through a lot since then. I moved just a smidge. I tried so hard not to move, but it was next to impossible.

I looked at him and said, "Did you get the sample?" He said he got a small sample. He hoped it was enough. It turns out, it was. After I got dressed and he came back in, he explained to me, if this doesn't work, the only other way to get this information is to crack my chest open to get that biopsy. I'm like, "WHAT? Crack my what??" Well, now the pain didn't seem so bad anymore. "Dr. E. let's go back in there and do it one more time just to make sure you got what you needed. We can have someone hold me down just for good measure."

He said very seriously, "No, we can't disturb the site."

"JEEZ, well if you put it that way. UGH. HOLY SHIT. What is going on here? He didn't really say crack my chest open, did he? Mumble mumble mumble FACE PLANT (?)

Our next step was to see the oncologist, Dr. W. He came highly recommended and was given all my tests, so he could create my treatment plan. He had reviewed all the data and would now be able to tell us what our next course of action should be or so I thought.

Now this part I will never ever forget. Jere and my mom are sitting to my left, and the good doctor is facing us. He's talking and talking. It just sounds like mumbling at first kind of like what the teacher in the Peanuts cartoon sounds like. "Waaaah, waah, waaah, waaah, waaah—faraway words that are completely unrecognizable to me. I wasn't even sure I'd heard part of what he was saying ... until I finally did. It was like, suddenly, I zero in on what this guy is saying, or has said, since he now seems to be done talking. At that moment, my eyes sharpened, and I zeroed in on him again. He's through talking, but I am just catching up. That's when I heard him saying that the biopsy Dr. E. had done had shown that my cancer has Stage IV.

My cancer, I hear him saying, is all over my mediastinum area, which consists of my whole left breast and around my nipple, my mammary glands, my chest, the left ventricle of my heart, my left lung, the whole side of my neck, my esophagus, and too many to even count lymph nodes. It's bad. I have a big hill to climb, you see.

This may sound crazy, but as I heard those words and my eyes came back into focus that day, a switch flipped in me, and I don't think it will ever switch back. Since that very moment I am different inside. My personality is different. It's strange and difficult to explain, but the chemical balance that had always been a part of me, made me who I was, got scrambled or electrocuted or something, and I was no longer the same Viki I'd been for forty- four years. It was crazy, but a different me left that room that day and never came back. Weird!

I understand that it must be very difficult to have to do some of the things this doctor has to do. Today, indeed, I understand so much more than I did then but then, wow, not so much at all. Because of all that was going through my mind, all I heard was blathering on and on about how he had consulted with this doctor and that doctor, and they all had come to the same conclusion. It was simple: There was nothing they could do for me. He was very sorry. But I should probably go home and get my affairs in order.

Wait, WHAT?! Had I just heard him, right? What had he said? Mom and Jere were crying to my left, and something just snapped inside me. I pretty much lunged across the room and grabbed the good doctor by his shirt collar. I'm not a violent person, and I didn't grab him in a violent manner, but I did grab him a bit aggressively. I needed him to look me in the eye. I needed him to really see me.

Viki. A person. A human being. ME.

"YOU DIDN'T CONSULT ME!" I shrieked. "You talk about consulting this doctor and that doctor, but you didn't consult me! What about what I have to say? *I don't care what you have to cut off! I don't care what you stick in me!* I will take ANYTHING. Pain, needles, medicine, I don't care how much pain you cause me. I'm a MOM! I want to raise my children. Don't you understand? I'M GOING TO BE THE ONE. I'm going to make it! I'm going to be that one person!"

Then I went quiet. The room was quiet, too, and no one said a word for a good minute until finally the doctor began to speak. "Okay, how about we start with chemotherapy treatment first? If your tumors shrink, then we can talk about a mastectomy, alright?"

"Okay," I said, my voice no longer shrieking. Ironically, soon after that meeting with Dr. W., I ran into Dr. E, and I knew he would tell me the truth. I looked at him and said, "Am I going to make it to Dell's bar-mitzvah?"

He quietly said, "No, no, you're not."

You know that was a real kick in the teeth, but I went home, wrote out the deposit check for a party venue we liked, drove straight over there, and handed them the check.

Undoubtedly, at that moment, these doctors knew then something that I didn't know. They knew that I would most likely die of congestive heart failure before I would die from the cancer. But what they didn't know was ME. They didn't know who I was as a person. They didn't know my strength, my perseverance, and my full determination to kick cancer. They didn't know there was no way I was leaving my children! NO FREAKING WAY!

So that left me with only one option: FIGHT FIGHT FIGHT LIKE HELL. So that's what I did. I promised God that when I got through all this, then it would be my turn to help. That is why I have dealt with all this pain. Because I got to raise my kids, it's my turn now. It has been such a heavy burden on my heart that these ten years while I have been living, all those other sick women have died.

Since I Am the One, now, I must give back to God.

Since I Am the One, now, I must save women.

Now, so far, so good.

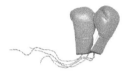

Chemotherapy Chapter

I approached chemotherapy with the fierce determination of a drill sergeant. I liken it to tunnel vision. I had no room for any noise. I was driven forward in one direction, and that was to concentrate on my recovery. I was really only capable of communicating with my children because they and my immediate family needed me desperately. It is difficult to describe how focused I was, but I knew that my life was hanging in the balance. I had my "One Job," and failure was out of the question!! Those perfect children needed me, and they were so little. Just the thought of someone else raising them made me want to throw up! I wasn't going to let that happen.

That's why thinking like that was dangerous.

I no longer left any room for such thoughts. My tunnel vision focused my direction sharply on one and one thing only, and that one thing was HEALING. Unfortunately, sometimes

I look back, and I realize I must have appeared angry. But never confuse anger for focus because that just wasn't the case. I know it may seem strange to some, but honestly, I never really felt anger—not even at the beginning when it would have been a fair response and very appropriate to cry and say "Why me?". I never did or said that either.

I know you are probably thinking, okay, this girl is lying or a real Pollyanna, but the plain fact is that from the very beginning even when I didn't know the dire situation I was in, I just was focused on the what's next. What can I do to get better? How do I make it right? From the beginning, I just focused on my future. What can I say, I had tunnel vision from the start. I'm a mom first and always and will always put my babies first!!! I wasn't wrong because, according to my doctor, I didn't have a lot going for me. I had my work cut out for me, and I needed all my concentration, all my strength, and all my tunnel vision and laser focus.

On my first day of chemotherapy, I was armed with the most wonderful green velour blanket my mom bought for me. She does her research as well, and she was told that I would get very cold. I appreciated her research and her beautiful green velour blanket because the minute the needle entered my vein and they released my medication it was like ice entering my veins, sending instant shivers through my entire body. So, yes, I was very grateful for mom's comforting green velour blanket. Then, fortunately that was about the time they slipped me a mickey, and I fell thankfully asleep through the worst of it.

Chemotherapy was grueling, long, and arduous. Each week it would build and build, and I would get sicker and weaker and paler. It became more and more challenging. The very high doses of steroids I was taking for other problems created side effects that conflicted with the effects of the chemo. I was puffy from the steroids but pale and flaxen skinned from the chemo. My appetite was all over the map. The steroids made me hungry, but the chemo made me sick and nauseous. I was a mess. There were lots of mood swings and bouts of fatigue. It was a very confusing time. It took all my concentration to keep my patience and calm around the children. That, in turn, sapped so much energy that I barely had any patience and calm for the kids. Do you see the cycle?

I had to learn to navigate food differently because I could tolerate only certain foods. I would settle on carbs.

That was about the only thing I could digest. There's a misnomer that no one really knows about breast cancer and women. We associate cancer and great weight loss. While that may be true for many cancers, there's some evidence that the opposite could be true for most breast cancer cases. Yep, women with breast cancer are at a higher risk of gaining weight during treatment. It's a big problem. This can cause depression, which in turn can affect some people's will to fight the disease or just properly take care of themselves. A simple thing like weight gain can lead to so many other complications. It's scary and hidden in the cancer world or any world for that matter. The more women's discussion groups there are, the more it's becoming clear that it's a common problem. But there's not enough of that to have any sort of data written on the subject, at least not that I have seen.

Chemotherapy droned on, and I kept right on with it. The nurses at the clinic were— and still are—fabulous. I'm not sure if I have mentioned this before because I suppose it's sort of a sensitive subject for me—the bell they have in the chemotherapy lobby. You see I was going to suggest that these amazing nurses should get to ring that bell every damn day. They are true heroes. But I need to reference the significance of the bell. When a chemotherapy patient has completed treatment and is considered in remission, they get to ring the bell for all to hear. It's a very proud moment. The whole floor claps. Alas, I will never ring that bell because my treatment never ends. One could look at that two ways; at least I'm here and getting treatment or sometimes a tiny little bit of pettiness might drop in and you just want to ring the goddamn fuckin' bell. But that's just a few grumpy moments. The nurses are on their feet running constantly, and they are educated and very knowledgeable. They have earned their stripes; that is for sure. They must find their job very rewarding because I think it is a thankless job quite often which really ticks me off. I believe they do it for us, the patients.

I know I'm so grateful for them every day. I try to show my gratitude in any way I can. Sometimes it's difficult because we are just so sick, but we remember their voices or the touch of their hands and their kindness. If I was taken by ambulance, for example, and wasn't fully myself, I always come back to a hospital and try and say, thank you to those that took care of me while I couldn't care for myself. I think it's important. Because as I said, it's a thankless job, so who's going to thank them if not us.

I did learn some lessons, however, and that was not everyone was caring and kind. There were some experiences I had that were so upsetting that they will stay with me for the rest of my life. I think mostly because I was so sick, it left such a profound stamp on me that someone could be so cruel to someone like me that was at her worst and most vulnerable state. It just baffles me still today looking back. I'm babbling. Let me tell you the story.... I like to be prepared in advance.

You may have figured this out about me already. I'm a five-steps-ahead kind of girl. Given that fact, I wanted to make sure I had the most perfect wig ready to go when my hair fell out because I wanted a seamless transition. Johns Hopkins had this wig department that was upscale and could do anything for you. It sounded right up my alley. The three amigos (Mom, Jere, and I) headed straight for the wig shop. We met up with the head honcho, and she was very nice (that day); we tried on all kinds of wigs. I was able to get a wig with real hair, but it was very expensive. I had no idea what went into all of this— what a production. I wanted to have highlights in the wig just like my own hair and so forth. She said that was no problem; that would be done after I chose the wig and matched the color of my hair. After we selected the wig, we put down a deposit, and off we went.

It took quite a while for the wig to come in, and my hair was falling out rapidly, so I was glad for my process of always thinking ahead. When we went in to collect the wig, I was disappointed. It didn't look anything like I thought it would. It didn't have the highlights in it. The color didn't match. For all that money, I was very upset, and now we were running out of time. Wig lady said, "Don't worry. I'll send it back and get you a new one. It won't take long."

It was weeks before the replacement wig came in, and I was still not happy. When we three amigos went to pick it up, it was the same exact wig that we returned in the first place. I thought I was going to have a nervous breakdown.

HELLO, WIG LADY. ARE YOU HIGH? THIS IS THE SAME GOD DAMN WIG!!! Then the snide came out in the wig lady. It must have been underneath all along; we just were too busy to notice. You know, like when someone farts, and the smell takes a while to get to you? Well, the fart just got to us, and boy, did it stink! Her lips started to curl, and she just looked at us and said, "I told you it would look like this. I'm not sending another perfectly good wig back, and you are responsible for the cost for this wig."

I said, "Where are the highlights?"

She said, "Well, you have to put them in."

ARE YOU FREAKING KIDDING ME? WE JUST ASKED YOU THAT SAME QUESTION WHEN THE LAST WIG CAME IN, AND YOU SAID IT WAS AN ERROR. NOW ALL OF A SUDDEN, IT'S A DIFFERENT STORY. WELL, WHICH IS GOING TO STICK TO THE WALL TODAY?

Oh, she was so rude. You all should have seen her—so self-righteous. She was actually going to charge us more to put highlights and cut the wig. I couldn't believe it. She was going to do that all along. She charged us a small fortune for the wig and was always going to charge us that back-end fee, and never was clear about that. I wonder how she sleeps at night. We can't be the only suckers she has done this to.

She has a shop right in the middle of the hospital. It's like a business for those poor, unwitting victims filing in like lambs to be slaughtered. As long as, Johns Hopkins doesn't do anything about it, she will remain the rip-off artist to unassuming, desperate, sick, and sad people and take advantage of them repeatedly as she did to me. (We wrote a letter of complaint to Johns Hopkins and never received a response back.)

Back to my story of where I was going with my feelings about how my hair was now falling out. (I just want to interrupt myself again here and tell you that story first because it was so pivotal in my cancer journey.) I was losing my beautiful hair, little by little. I would wake up in the morning, and there would be chunks of my hair on my pillow. That would be so startling to me, such a very upsetting way to wake up, let me tell you! Then I would be so afraid to run a brush through my hair, or God forbid SHOWER! After my shower, I would be sweeping up my hair for about thirty minutes. It would not only set me back in getting out of the house, if I had an appointment or such, but again it was very unnerving.

I can't quite explain how I was feeling, but nothing up to that point or even really after was so upsetting to me as watching my hair fall out. It was like losing a little part of myself each day; it was slowly breaking my heart. At the time I don't think I realized it, but I knew I couldn't continue to sweep these huge piles of hair up every day. So, I called my friend and longtime hair consultant for advice. She opened her shop on a Sunday just for privacy. When Isabella asked to come, I didn't think. I agreed to let her join me, and off we went. That's my greatest regret today. I had no real idea of what was boiling down inside me and how sensitive I was about my hair. When my lovely and ever-so-kind friend gently and lovingly shaved the remaining locks from my head, tears streamed down my face, and I just couldn't control them. Even as I write this, tears are running down my cheeks. What is it about the hair? I wrote something at the time so poignant that I will share it today because I could never explain better. It's a loss of hair—loss of self. I look in the mirror, and I don't see myself. It's not as if it's bad, but I don't feel like myself.

Losing my hair was a huge deal. I'd never realized how much I identified with my hair. So much so that when I lost it, I couldn't look at myself in the mirror. I was ashamed. I didn't want to face my friends or family. You can never really prepare for what chemo will do to you. It made me feel so sick. My shoulder-length, straight, thick hair kept falling out and out and out. I needed to get that broom to sweep up the bathroom every morning. The constant shedding got to be too difficult, so I went to my trusted hair stylist on a Sunday when the shop was closed (as I earlier mentioned) to shave off the remaining strands of my hair. I had no idea just how emotional it would be for me, so when she asked, I allowed my sweet daughter to join me. Big mistake.

When my hair was shaved, tears just rolled down my face. No matter how hard I tried, I just couldn't keep them from falling. My daughter was rubbing my leg and telling me how beautiful I looked. My eight-year -old daughter. It is a memory I don't enjoy recalling. Yes, I had a beautiful wig to wear (which is a long story in itself) and felt okay with it on. But from that day on .... even still today... I don't see the same woman in the mirror. I remember my husband's face when he saw me when I returned home. It was that split-second look of horror before he could put his game face on. My son gave me that same look.

From that day, my son and daughter never wanted me to leave the house without my wig on. As time passed, I didn't care so much anymore, and the wig was itchy, but my children felt better when I wore it. My Bella would say, "Mommy, are you going to wear your wig when you come to my school? Mommy, if my friend so and so comes over, will you wear your wig?"

So today, even though my hair has grown back— curly! —I still don't see Viki in the mirror staring back. It's not as if I hate the person I see; it's more as if I'm resigned to the person I see. My mom asks me why don't I cut my hair short and spiky like when it was first growing in? It looked so cute and contemporary then she remarketed. I know it looks more like a mullet now or something out of a Vegas show in the Elvis days, but I "NEED" it back at shoulder length. Somehow, I get back control then. If I want to cut it off at that point, at least it'll be on my own terms.

I'm in control, not cancer. But I wonder when it's shoulder-length again, will I look like me again? I fear not. Certainly, there is the possibility that I will never get that long hair again because my diseases will return, and I'll lose all my hair again... but mostly I fear that the person I'm looking for in the mirror is gone.

I realize it doesn't have to be bad to be different, but when you are used to something for forty plus years, it takes more than a year to grow accustomed to someone else when you look in the mirror.

In addition to my hair, I had a beat-up arm. I say arm because I could only use one arm. To this day and always, I can't use blood pressure cuffs or have needle sticks of any kind on my left arm. I believe it has to do with my not having much of a lymphatic system and not being able to protect myself or absorb or cleanse my body properly. Soon it was getting difficult to find a vein to administer my chemo treatments. It would take a long time to find one, and then that one would blow out and we would have to start all over again. It was quite grueling, and my arm looked very sad. So I'm stuck with one ugly looking sorry excuse for an arm. It became more and more difficult as the months marched on. My poor arm struggled to maintain a healthy vein throughout the treatment.

Finally, four months passed, and my chemotherapy treatment had come to an end. I was left exhausted, nauseous, and black and blue. Now came the real test. According to Dr. J., I needed to have at least a ninety-eight to a ninety-nine percent result, which as you can imagine, was going to be tough to reach especially with my statistics. It was back to the waiting game all over again. The nerves came back, the pacing began, and Mom, Jere, and I all began our round robin of worry.

Before I move forward, I think I need to do one more of my famous backward slides to clarify some of my journey. You'll understand more as I go on, and I think you will appreciate that I stopped and moved back even though I know it was a very exciting part of my life story. In due time folks, in due time. Anyway, when I was first diagnosed and realized, I knew I was going to have to do a lot of research. I called an old friend, Dr. J., who used to live in Harrisburg and worked at the Hershey Medical Center in the pediatric radiology department and now was living in Indiana running his own center. One of the reasons I reached out to Dr. J. was that he was working with a different type of radiation called proton radiation rather than the radiation that Johns Hopkins was going to use and that most people are familiar with as photon radiation. The difference is that proton radiation is more targeted—it can go around the organs (thereby saving the organs) and stop on a dime. Photon radiation, on the other hand, has a lot of splatter and covers a large area at a time without being able to control it as well. This is a problem for me for two reasons; first it goes in through the front and out through the back, and second the scatter couldn't be controlled; for both reasons my organs would be badly damaged beyond repair. Because of where my cancer and my tumors were, this means that the photon radiation would do a lot of damage, and I would probably die of congestive heart failure. Dr. J. asked me to send my x-rays for his review.

Not long after I sent the x-rays, we were having long, extensive phone conversations. Much to my good fortune, this longtime friend was well-versed in this area and really was concerned about my x-rays and was desperately trying to see a way out of my predicament.

The next thing I knew, Mom, Jere, and I were sitting around my kitchen table because Dr. J. had flown in and was going over a plan he had for us—a very thin plan. He tells us that if I get a ninety-eight to ninety-nine percent positive response from the chemo treatment, (which isn't exactly an easy thing to do, you understand) that would be the first necessary MUST in his plan. A positive response means that my huge tumor must shrink by ninety-eight to ninety-nine percent. It was practically unheard of! He looked grim about the prospects of that happening, but I didn't!! This was the first crack I'd had so far, and I was going to turn it into a hole and then a crater if I had to. I can work with a crack. Oh, yeah, this could work. If for some blessing that happens, then when you get your radical mastectomy, you must remain flat. You can't expand the expanders. Point of reference: They put expanders in place in your chest to try and keep what's left of your breast tissue stretched so they can use it later for some sort of reconstruction. But my chest wall was so badly damaged, and now my chances for anything were slim. As far as I was concerned, that was the least of my worries. From there then he would try mapping me for proton radiation therapy, but there are a lot of ifs in between; he kept reminding me. Yes, I understand, I said. Then he left and said he would keep in touch.

Now you see why Mom, Jere, and I were on pins and needles

waiting for the results of the chemotherapy. My life was literally hanging in the balance. The next part is just not to be believed. If I wasn't there, I wouldn't have believed it myself. We received word that my test results had come in. We were to head back to Johns Hopkins to get the news, but Dr. W. apparently wasn't available to discuss it with me. Instead, his right-hand Nurse Practitioner N. was to give us the news. It made me wonder if the news was going to be bad and he was afraid I would choke him again. NP N. called us into her office. We looked up, anxiously waiting for the ax to fall, and she started going on and on about things I had no idea what she was talking about.

Our anxiety was rising quickly, and just when I was about to interrupt her and ask her to cut to the chase, the phone rang. I'm thinking, "There is no way she is going to pick up the phone. I mean we are in the middle of a life and death conversation." Boy, was I wrong She picked up the phone; it was her husband. When I realized it was a personal call, I knew she wouldn't be unprofessional in a meeting, such as this one especially with my LIFE IN THE BALANCE. I gave her far too much credit; oh, yes, I did. We could hear her loudly and clearly on the phone as we were sitting there in that small little office, astonished, open mouthed, frozen. She was acknowledging that her husband had his car broken down (poor fellow; It's not like he was dying or anything like that), and he needed her help in arranging a tow truck and picking him up at such and such time and on and on ... blah. blah. While we are waiting for news that could save my life. ARE YOU FUCKING KIDDING ME! GET THE FUCK OFF THE PHONE!!!! But I was a lady today. I didn't strangle anyone. I think that's why Dr W pawned me off onto NP. N to begin with, so I was getting a reputation. Finally, she ends the conversation all flighty and says, "Sorry, that couldn't be helped."

We looked at her in unison and said let's cut to the chase. What are my results? We have waited long enough, and we have no idea what you were talking about before. What is my number? What did I do already? She said, "Oh", with that little hand over her mouth, "Sorry, you did great." What's great? "Your tumor is gone. There's a one to two percent margin left. That's it. It's remarkable. We've never seen anything like it before. You are cleared to go onto the next phase and get your mastectomy."

Holy shit, Hot damn, Whew, One down. My tunnel vision wouldn't allow me to over celebrate, but I did close my eyes, blow out a deep breath, thank God, and give myself a quiet minute of thankfulness before buckling back down again. Mom and Jere were still celebrating and didn't notice the sharp look that had come back into my eyes; my new determination and goals took over.

As some smells can take you back to experiences, so can others, today whenever I'm getting my maintenance chemotherapy treatments, I can hear the click, click, click of her heels coming down the hall, and it just sends shivers right down my spine. click, click, click, click, click, click, click ...

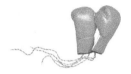

Mastectomy Chapter

After much deliberation, I chose a surgeon for my mastectomy. She was tough, too. She wanted to know if I lost all use of my arm during surgery, would I be ok with that? Would I still want the surgery? Oh yes, let's put this into perspective here. Hmm, do I want to die, or do I want my arm? Tough decision, but I'll go with door number two and choose to live. Duh!!! Then even though it was premature, I chose my plastic surgeon because she was going to come into the end of the surgery and place the expanders. I mentioned the expanders before. They are placed to try and stretch the skin and keep it taut for when the time comes for some sort of reconstruction. However, they were placing my expanders but not inflating them because Dr. J. said he needs for me to remain flat.

The day of the surgery I was—I'm not sure what; I was losing a part of me that I've had all my life. Personally, I wasn't overly fond of them, but they were mine, and I was territorial all of the sudden. This was a bit surprising to me and didn't make sense, but nothing was making any sense these days. I had Jere take pictures of my breasts the night before my surgery just in case Isabella wants to know why she looks like this, or I want to look back and remember. I just thought it prudent. To this day, I haven't looked yet, but I've thought about it.

I was warned that the surgery was going to be very long and complicated. In fact, they were concerned with how long it may become and about having to close me up before it's complete because I'll have been under too long. Dr J. (not the Dr. J. that's doing my radiation) is also a J. SHE is the surgeon doing my mastectomy. After I'm prepped for surgery, she comes in my cubicle to make sure all is well before she goes to scrub up. Then she drops a bomb on me and continues to say unfortunately, it's just bad luck, but she has some sort of seminar out of the county and must leave immediately after my surgery. She won't be around for my post op care, but not to worry I will be in great hands. Her best resident will be taking over my case.

From that moment on, just about everything went (how do I sum this up) from good to bad or as I refer to it as Fucked Up! The surgery itself went ok as surgeries go, I guess. It went too long, so Dr. M. (my plastic surgeon that came in at the end and placed the expanders) was correct with her concern about the surgery length. What tends to happen in these instances is the surgeon goes in like a bull in a china shop, and the plastic surgeon then comes in and has to clean everything up before she can get down to her own business, so it takes her twice as long, and therefore, time runs out.

That is what happened in my case, as she explained it to me. I was under about eleven hours for this surgery, and after everything my body had already been through, that was more than she wanted to risk me being under anesthesia, so she closed me up without doing some of the things she wanted to do and saved them for a future procedure.

After a lengthy stay in recovery, I'm wheeled to my private room which I'm told I'm very fortunate to receive. (Who did I have to kill to get this room?) I was placed on the V.I.P. floor at Hopkins called Marburg. My first memory was of crying out in pain as they transferred me from bed to bed. My Mom and Jere, close behind, grimacing in residual pain. I think a nurse appeared to introduce herself, but I can't be quite sure given the circumstances. While Jere and Mom hovered over me, they hooked me up to a morphine pump which I didn't want and told me to push the button with my thumb every 15 minutes or as needed. To my horror, the nurse then proceeded to put her finger on my thumb and push it on the medication button and released the morphine into my system. I don't like Morphine; I was pissed, but I was also exhausted and in pain.

The theme was taking shape quickly. I was left alone; we couldn't get a nurse or anyone to pay any kind of attention to me. My room was a pigsty. There was garbage everywhere. I don't even know where the trash came from, but I just remember the trash can was overflowing, and there was garbage all over the floor. I couldn't move; not without any sort of assistance, that's for sure. My body had just been through a major surgery, and I couldn't even lift my tush up for a bedpan—not that I could find a nurse to help me with that either. Now I was lying in my own pee; it was gross. Finally, a nurse would come in to wipe me off, give me a bedpan, and leave right away, but not before she would push my damn thumb down on that morphine. Finally, I had it with that and made my mom unplug me from the machine—no more morphine for me. Meantime, the whole time I am on this "VIP" floor sitting in my urine-soaked bed, in my garbage filled room, on this fancy floor with the polished wood floors, a young girl keeps circling up and down the hall for crying out loud and handing out little cucumber sandwiches on a silver tray offering them to Jere and my Mom as if they are at some kind of a cocktail party. If I wasn't there, I wouldn't believe it myself. Truly unbelievable.

Now if this wasn't enough of a nightmare, then I guess I just wasn't thinking big enough because along came Dr. Resident. Boy, was he everything that Dr. J. promised he would be and more. If he was her best resident, then she has a really crappy department!! This guy didn't have the credentials, at least not in my opinion, to be a vet—let alone the bedside manner to be a doctor.

I was in a tangle of nerves and stress from the moment he came into my room. He was horrible. He must have suffered from some kind of abuse by someone somewhere in his life for him to treat others this way. He was an awful little man and mean. Who would be mean to a woman with stage 4 metastatic cancer that had just gone through four months of chemotherapy treatment and had a eleven-hour radical mastectomy? I ask you what kind of human being treats another human, especially one so damaged, like that? I think he was deriving pleasure from it. We told him that the nurses haven't been to my room; they haven't even tried to get me out of bed. I explained to him, please help me, I'm lying here in my urine, and my room is filled with trash. Look around. Can't you see what's going on here? He looked at me and actually ignored my question. He didn't look around the room or care that I was living in garbage. He wasn't even concerned as my doctor that I had been lying for hours in my own urine, and no one had come in to try to get me out of bed to try and help me move just a bit. I was totally immobile.

He simply looked at me and said, "I'm going to discharge you today."

I said," What? Are you nuts? I can't walk. Get your staff to do their job and help me start moving so I can go to the bathroom myself; then maybe we can talk about discharge, but I'm clearly in no shape to be discharged.

Are you nuts?"

He just started walking away and said, "Well, we discharge all mastectomy patients around this time."

Like you can put us all in one box and treat us all the same because Lord knows I'm sure the procedures are all the same as someone with stage one or stage two cancer. I mean a radical mastectomy that took eleven hours that had to be closed before they completed surely does not seem the same as someone with a four-hour stage one procedure. By all means treat us all the same and hope by hell you won't get yourself sued when the patient suffers from a huge infection, you moron!! Furthermore, do your job!! How can you release a patient knowing she hasn't been properly cared for by the nursing staff. Knowing that patient hasn't been taken out of the bed once, taken to the bathroom, exercised, or walked or anything. With all that information, this doctor is coming into my room now, at this point, probably every thirty minutes harassing me and trying to tell me if I don't leave, he's going to call security. Can you believe the audacity of the man? And Hopkin's let him get away with it.

We wrote a letter about our experience on this "V.I.P." floor and our experience with Dr. J's. protege Resident. Johns Hopkins disappointedly did nothing, not even a well-deserved apology. That was disrespectful to us and all we'd been through and all the faith we'd put into Hopkins up to that point and continued to do afterward. It was disrespectful of them. If you can now picture this, I can't move; I'm lying in my own urine soaked mattress, the room now has double the garbage all over the floor, and this young girl keeps coming around with these stupid cucumber sandwiches that's becoming so annoying you just want to throw the whole stupid tray at her and say, would you just pick up a fucking broom and drop the goddamn sandwiches that no one wants. What we really want is the fucking garbage out of my room and the pee out of my bed. Do you think maybe you could handle that???

Then, of course, thirty minutes are up, and Dr. Obnoxious himself comes back into my room to threaten me some more. I'm sure there are laws against this sort of thing, and I'm sure I had rights to kick his ass out of my room, but you have to understand, I was weaker than I have ever been. I was really in bad shape. My Mom and Jere were furious but didn't want to upset me because I was getting increasingly upset. Dr. Obnoxious was really starting to get on my very last nerve to the point where I was getting really agitated. When I get agitated, I become immovable. I made a decision, and that was final. I need peace and tranquility to heal, and I wasn't getting it here. There were very bad vibes in the air, and I did not like the direction this was going. I got where I got because of positive and uplifting thoughts and a lot of perseverance. I wasn't about to let this little, little man (because that's what he was a "little" man) get in my way. There was NO chance of that. I wouldn't let anyone get in my way; let alone this weasel.

I asked Jere to call for a wheelchair. (By this time, it was around 8:30 at night.) We walked or wheeled out of the hospital right then and there. We didn't check out; I didn't change out of my gown; I merely took a pillow to clutch against my chest for the pain, and off we went. See ya. Wouldn't want to be ya!! No one said a word. That nightmare stayed with me for a very long time.

From there we headed to a hotel. Jere stayed with Mom and me for the night, and when he saw we were okay, he left for Harrisburg and left me in Mom's capable hands to recuperate until I was well enough for the drive back to Harrisburg. Boy, was she capable, alright. A tough taskmaster. She had me up and out of that bed every hour to see how much I could walk the halls of the hotel. At first, I could barely make it to our door, but the more she pushed me, I started to get further and further. She should have been a nurse. She would have been terrific. We spent a week in that hotel room. We had a much better time together, and moods began to change other than the occasional moodiness of constant pain. We watched movies, ate junk food, walked, took naps, walked, ate junk food, walked.... You get the idea. Finally, we hit the road for the big burg. I still wasn't feeling great, but I was doing a hell of a lot better. I still had the pillow we swiped from the hospital which I needed to hold close and protect my chest. Well, one thing led to another and as I tend to do, I started getting very nauseous and carsick more and more until finally I'm vomiting into that pillow I brought from the hospital. How ironic! Well, of course, this is the one-time Mom doesn't have her bucket and paper towels. Now, she is gagging as well, which is tricky because she's reacting to the smell. She's driving and gagging and trying to pull over (yikes) and finally gets over to a gas station... She gets out, and I'm pretty sure she threw up. (OH MY!) Then she helps me into the gas station to clean up, and we get back in the car and leave. We leave the pillow on the side of the road because it's leaking vomit. I think that's a good reason. For the longest time every time we drove to Hopkins, we would see that pillow on the side of the road. (Mom and I think that's so funny. We burst out giggling every time we see that pillow!)

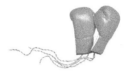

Indiana Chapter

Literally three weeks after my mastectomy and a month after the completion of my four months of chemo, Dr. J. wanted me on a plane to the Indiana University's Health Proton Therapy Center located in Bloomington. As Dr. J. had carefully explained to me, this was the only proton therapy in the U.S. to use a uniform-scanning beam for dose delivery which decreases undesirable neutron dose to patients. The center had opened in 2004 and actually closed in 2014. I understood very little about the Institute, but I did understand it was a life preserver being thrown to me, and I was determined to grab it. I also understood that once I arrived in Bloomington, Dr. J. spent something like 270 hours mapping me for radiation treatment. Probably, the longest case he's ever spent on. YIKES. All I could offer him was my pledge: 'I'm worth it, D.J. I promise you. I'm a really good patient. I'll do everything you say. I'll hold really still, and I'm going to survive, so I won't be a waste of your time. I know it!"

Now, just to let you all know it wasn't easy getting transferred into Dr. J.'s care. First, I had to get released from my very important hospital and convince them that Dr. J. could do better for me in this one area. Dr. J., God bless him, called and not only spoke to the radiologist but also to Dr. W., and they consulted as they do a lot, and both agreed that I was better off in Dr. J.'s care for my radiation treatment. (My research paid off big time.) Anyway, I would return to Johns Hopkins when my radiation was complete, but that was going to be at least four months down the road. Now Dr. W. made an agreement with me that I would get all my chemotherapy treatment done at Johns Hopkins. In other words, I was not to transfer my cocktail to my local hospital as most people do. He said my case was far too aggressive, and if he were to remain my doctor, I was to remain at Johns Hopkins, so I stayed. What was so amazing during this time, he was willing to transfer my chemotherapy treatment to a hospital in Indiana because chemotherapy for me never ends. I am what you call a "lifer". My hard chemo was completed, and now I moved into my maintenance stage of chemo which I will remain until God-willing whenever forever is?

The next obstacle was my insurance company. Ever since I was diagnosed, that issue has been nothing but a fight. I thought fighting the cancer was going to be my toughest obstacle, but I didn't know it would be a tossup in comparison to fighting the insurance company. I sure didn't have much strength in me for that fight as well, but I was determined not to bankrupt my family. The insurance company kept saying I was doing an experimental treatment; I was doing no such thing. Proton radiation had been around for quite some time and had been used in brain cancer and prostate cancer on a regular basis. Who is to say it can't be used in my case if a doctor is willing to map me? Well, it got continually denied.

Since I was to leave for treatment in Indiana in about a week, I was running out of time. My divorced parents, who never talk to one another, were both willing to put up their homes so I could get this treatment done. It would have cost around $400,000 to $500,000. That's a lot of money for one treatment, and who knows what lay ahead? Finally, I was desperate. I just couldn't let my parents put up their homes. Just that thought made me sicker. So, I got creative and sent flowers to the secretary of the medical director of the insurance company (Let me tell you it was no easy feat finding out the name and phone number; they aren't just lying around listed.) When she called to thank me for the flowers, she let me tell her my whole story and said she would take it to the director. I was so very grateful. Soon after that, I got my insurance approval.

Thus, three weeks after my mastectomy, my mom and I were on a plane to Indiana. That was not easy. I looked like hell, a complete train wreck, as I was wheeled to the plane's entrance. But there was no time for me to think about how I felt. Mom and I had a lot to do while we were there and not a lot of time to do it in. Not only did we have to take care of all the doctor stuff, but we had to find us a place to live for the next four months. It had to be close by the facility as well as furnished and large enough for my family to visit. After all, it was close to summer break, and my kids would be through with school in about a month. I wanted and needed them to be with me for the entire summer.

As Dr. J. patiently showed me around the facility, I tried to grasp exactly what would be happening to me here. Wow, they were going to strap me onto this narrow table and hoist me up very high in the air (Bear in mind I don't even like rollercoasters, and this was far higher) and direct a pointy beam straight at me—like something out of "Star Trek." Very science fiction. Very scary! Next, they took all these plaster models of my head and face. The kind of model's actors take for horror movies to enhance the monster character of the moment. That was eerily creepy. I didn't have much energy to begin with, but, boy, was I wiped out when those models were all done. The precision with which he measured so carefully and mathematically. They say you don't use math outside of school; well, here they sure do, wow. I just can't imagine the time and attention it took for him to devote to my mapping. I now realized the behind- the scenes multitude of hours he spent on my behalf. I'll be forever grateful to this man.

Mom and I had the next exhausting task of looking for a place for us all to live. Now if it were just for us, it would have been a much easier operation, but I wanted to bring the kids and Jere out, and why not damn it, so mom and I set about making my dream come true. We figured we would need three bedrooms, furnished and for only about four months, not an easy feat. My energy by now was next to nil as we set out to look in the neighborhood. We had about three places on our list. The first place was yucky. That made us nervous right away.

The second place only had two bedrooms, but it was a very nice place. We liked it, and we were really tired and started to get a bit punchy. When mom and I get punchy, look out. Oh, how silly and bit giggly in a very incoherent way we were quickly becoming. Look out now. Oh, my mom discovered a closet in the apartment. Now, you must understand you would have thought she found the messiah! She was so very proud of herself. "Look ...Viki, Hurry! Come quick. You have to see this; I found a perfect place for the children."

I'm like "Ok, Mom. Coming. Where the hell are you????" Holy Shit!!!! My very mostly proper mother in her seventy's is lying in the middle of a very, very long closet floor, with a very, very large smile on her face. I thought she went wacko for sure.

"Oh. my God! You need Help!!"

She says, "No. Look. See how long and deep this closet is? Ahh ... Yeah?? Don't you get it?? It's perfect for the kids."

"What the Fuck, Mom. You want to put my kids in the closet for the summer? Are you nuts?"

"Viki ..Look.. It's big. Measure."

And oh my, I did measure. My mother laid down, and I measured her length, and then we measured her again, and, damn, those peanuts probably would have had a ball in there. I helped her up; we sat down and thought about it rationally and said... We can't put the kids in a closet.

What the hell is wrong with us? Oh my God, we need food NOW. After nourishment and a more rational head, we hit another spot, itchy coach, yuck, and then found a place we settled on. Bless Mom, she insisted on covering the rent for the summer, a huge help since the rent was not cheap. Of course, I felt a bit like a burden, but I was very appreciative.

The following day we were back on a plane home bound to Harrisburg. While Dr. J. finished mapping and getting ready for my arrival, I got my ducks in a row and prepared for my arrival back to Indiana as well. Before I knew it, that time had passed. Mom and I were together again—back on a plane to Indiana. We rented a car again and headed to our new home in Bloomington. My Bestie (bless her heart) mailed all the extras for us that would make us more comfortable—the things that cost too much to send on the plane. So kind of her and so much appreciated. We, of course, had luggage bulging to the brim being the respectable woman that we were. Sick or not, treatment or not, we were always going to look our very best.

When we ended up at the apartment, it was a bit of a mess. Let's just say things weren't quite what we were used to, but when I sat on my bed and I sank to the floor, Mom and I just giggled. That really was the last straw after a very long day. When we were given the choice of cable or the bed, we quickly shut up and chose cable. I watched that damn cable all night long. I would just call on Mom in the morning for a pull out of bed. Hey, that's what family is for.

After mom and I got settled, we were welcomed into the home of Dr. J. and his family—my friend, his beautiful wife, and his two handsome and terrific boys. They lived just a mile or two down the road from where we settled. When we entered, it was funny to see that their home was in a bit of disarray at the time due to an unfortunate lice mishap, so everything was still in plastic bags. Somehow that made me feel relieved knowing someone as organized as she was had situations out of her control as well. Is it crazy that that immediately put me at ease? We had a lovely dinner of pizza and pasta and got some great information on the area with things to do, and we went back to our little apartment—me to my sunken bed.

When the two of us explored the town of Bloomington, we found all kinds of yummy places to eat along with all kinds of lovely places to shop. We were two peas in a pod. Back in the apartment, we sat on our couch and watched our favorite shows and shared our snacks. I think everyone should have the opportunity, maybe not to be sick, but to spend this kind of time alone with your mom. At this stage in my life, it was such a blessing. It's almost worth getting sick.

The treatment itself wasn't so terrible, but it did build up, and it did become grueling. The hardest part was that there were mostly young children in the waiting room, which in itself was so hard to see. That was because proton radiation is done mostly for brain cancer, and Dr. J. had been a pediatric doctor at Hershey Medical Center before he came to Bloomington. Lots of kids with brain cancer made it a pretty tough waiting room. Mom and I bought boxes and boxes of books and toys for the waiting room and always gave when we left as a thank you, continuing to send more boxes every Christmas. If you saw those children, you would send boxes as well. You just want to see them smile. They had to be put to sleep every time they went into the chamber because it was so high and scary, and they couldn't move in there. Because that summer was extremely hot, the system kept breaking down. They would work around the clock to repair whatever needed to be fixed. It was crucial; I had my treatment every day. The children would always get taken care of first, which I would insist upon, even if they didn't, but the children didn't always need to go every day as I did. Mom and I could get the call to go in at two am or midnight or five at night or three in the afternoon. We just would never really know. That made it a bit difficult to plan our day, but as time marched on and the treatment built up in my system, I grew more tired and suffered from burns, so we ventured out less and less.

Charm, comic relief, and endearing love burst through our door in the name of my sister, Jill. Boy, were we glad to see her!! The band was back together, baby!! We are a bit like the Three Stooges but clumsier. If you looked up that group, you would find a picture of the three of us. Jill hadn't been with us more than three minutes before she stopped up the toilet. (If you know my sister, there isn't a toilet she doesn't stop up.) But what she did next was not to be believed. For hours we hadn't been able to get the toilet working, and we were getting desperate. What happened then was so funny, but, oh my goodness, when I SAY YOU HAD TO BE THERE, you had to be there. Oh, I love my sister! She simply scooped everything she had put in the you know what if you know what I mean and put it in a plastic bag. Then, as we were driving away, she threw the bag into the dumpster. However, since she does not have a good aim, the bag just kind of hung there so every time we drove past the dumpster, we saw it hanging there, and we would break out in hysterics. Such fun, we would have over stupid things, but it was just so good to laugh! Since then, we have been taking girl trips every year. Whether it's just a week at the beach or a more extravagant trip to St. Kitts, we make it a priority to take our "Girls' TRIP", and we laugh from beginning to end. Belly laughs are our priority. Jill stayed a couple of weeks, and we had a great time with her. She sure made my treatment was fun and full of adventure. What's that song Julie Andrews sings, "A spoonful of sugar makes the medicine go down". That's my sister Jill.

Not long after, the caravan of Jere, the kids, and my dad all arrived. It was a revolving door. Jere drove out the long ten-hour drive with the kids, so we would no longer have the expense of the rental car. Following him (bless his heart) was my dad; then he would fly back then the following day. That way when Jere left with the children, Mom and I still had a vehicle. Everyone chipped in that summer.

I was a lucky girl to have so many people who loved and cared about my happiness. Go, Dad, you saved the day! Everyone in my family in one way or another pitched in and played his/her part in making my life so much easier—my cousins, my sister, my husband, my mother, and my father. When I say family, I include my Michelle, who has been my childhood friend since I was seven; I can't tell you enough about her.

But the best part that summer was that my kids were having a ball and were so cute to have around. Jere took three weeks off from work and stayed with us for that time and returned to Indiana whenever possible. We hired a sitter and signed the kids up at the local YWCA camp where at ages eleven and eight, they did all sorts of fun things. At the end of the summer, they had this great program with everyone doing the YMCA dance at the end. We got up and danced badly with everyone. Unfortunately, we have it on video, so it's burned into my memory because Jere makes fun of me with it quite often. You can see the image of me, bald, flat chested, sheet-white, misspelling YMCA. I mean, come on. I would blackmail me, too.

As my four months in Indiana wound down, I spent time at Dr J.'s house, often enjoying his family. Mom and I love them, and I will always love his wife. They were all so welcoming and fun to be around. We were honestly sad when we left them. They remain in our hearts forever even if we don't get to talk to them as much anymore. That family is very special to us, and we will always love them very much.

There are so many other memories of that time. When I first arrived for treatment and was hoisted up, I was a bit scared. But the guys that took care of me throughout my treatment months were always "my guys", and they had my back. Tears are running down my face as I write about them now. They were special. Men aren't built like these men are built. They changed me and made me a better human. I will remember their kind touch forever. When treatment is finally completed, you get to do this amazing thing: You ring a bell—like a bell for God to hear, or like the town crier. I wish I would have not been so rushed at the time and appreciated it more in the moment. It's something I think about now and again because as I mentioned before I'm what you call a "lifer"— meaning I get chemotherapy for my lifetime, which, of course I'm grateful for, but sometimes when I'm there for like my hundredth time and I hear another person ring her chemo bell because her treatment is complete, a little piece of my heart breaks. I just really want to ring that bell for some reason. I'm not sure why. Irrational it is because theoretically ringing it wouldn't be good for me, but sometimes rational doesn't play well with others.

Leaving Indiana was bittersweet. Mom and I packed up everything. When we pulled out, we stopped and took a picture. I still have that picture. It was a good memory, believe it or not, and that always surprises us. The kids had a ball. They still talk about it fondly. They want to go back and visit the area. Unfortunately, the center lost its funding in 2014 and is no longer there. Dr. J. and his family moved to Maryland where he went to work for NIH. We still would like to visit because we enjoyed the area, and the kids' memories were positive which makes me so happy. I worked so hard that summer to make it a fun time for the kids and not about my being sick. Now all these years later my daughter is looking into colleges, and she is considering going to school there because her memories were so positive. Mom and I rocked that summer. We kicked ass. I prayed that I made that summer easy for those children, but only time would tell. My daughter telling me she would love to go back, and visit means I did something right.

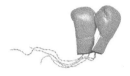

The Kids Chapter

When it was time to tell the children, they knew something was going on, but they were also kids worried about kid stuff which thank goodness is very normal. Jere and I sat them down on the floor. It was important to me first to get down to their level but in a non-threatening and very casual manner and then give them the truth. Always tell the truth, I believe it is very important. So knowing they had a very short attention span. I just said, "You know how Mommy and Daddy have been gone a lot? We have been going back and forth to a hospital in Maryland called Johns Hopkins, and Mommy has been getting a lot of medical tests. You understand what tests are, right?

"Pretty much."

"Good enough. Well, those tests told the doctors information about Mommy. I have cancer. Do you know what cancer is?"

"Yes, Mommy. Cancer is bad. My friend's mommy died from it. Are you going to die, Mommy? My friend's mom went bald. She looked weird. Are you going to look weird, too?"

"Ok, first things first. I'll tell you what; we will look at it this way. We all have jobs to do in this house, right?"

"Yes." (mumble)

"Ok, well, you both are responsible for doing your homework, getting good grades, making your beds every morning, helping out when needed, and most importantly (listen closely) having fun."

"Got it. Ok, Mom."

"Now it's Mommy's job to work hard and get better. You understand? That means it's my job, not yours. Ok? I got this, ok? Now you do your job, and I'll do mine, and that's how it works, right? I mean Daddy goes to work, and you don't go with him, and you don't try and clean teeth, right? So I'm good. Now one more thing. To answer your second question, yes, I will be bald. I will look very funny. I will look like something out of one of your crazy characters from one of those video games you love so much. But it will grow back and just think about all the jokes you guys can come up with in the meantime. Now go play." And off they went.

That day the kids were eleven and eight but probably with what they have gone through who knows how old they actually were. I've always thought about the road less traveled in the sense that the kids were on a certain trajectory (in life), and BAM this happens, changes them forever, and sends them on a splintered road in a different direction. I'll always wonder if

I made my children stronger, perhaps more independent, and send them down a road that will lead them to success, or will they be stuck in a rut forever, and it will be because the road changed, and maybe I will always feel somewhat responsible. It's something I think about quite a lot. I suppose it's my mother's baggage, and I carry quite a lot. You would think I was the Hunchback of Notre Dame.

Despite all odds Dell was a Bar-Mitzvah. Remember when I said I walked out of Dr W.'s. office a different Viki and said I never changed back, this is one of those examples of something the old Viki would NEVER do. I was so bold that whole day, the weekend really. Then I talked my family into doing a crazy surprise performance at the affair. Jere, Bella, and I all dressed in bright gold lame' outfits resembling Mc Hammer running out to a choreographed dance to *You Can't Touch This*.... You would have thought we were running out naked for the roar of the crowd. Everyone was so surprised; they loved it. Then Dell came out and did a fabulous break dance piece. It was so much fun no one even noticed that the ovens broke down and the meal was two hours late.

Things started to settle down more, if there was such a thing, but the kids, especially Dell, were really active in soccer. We were driving to tournaments all over the place, getting hotels, dragging coolers, tents, and a share of food (the team usually chipped in). Believe it or not most of the time it was pretty fun. We would also spend a good two—maybe more— weeks if I could get away with it at the beach. I called it my happy place.

Bella really is our beach girl. Dell, I think, likes to go but doesn't like the beach itself. It's strange. I think he just likes the vacation aspect. It goes back to his days of sensory issues. I think the beach is a trigger for him. But Bella likes it as much as I do. If I ever can afford a beach house, (unlikely) I'd leave it to her. She loves it. I love being able to give her some independence. Both kids love that. Dewey is really safe, and the place we stay is centrally located, so I allow the kids to go and get food and bring it back or walk around a bit. As they get older, that has expanded. Bella is seventeen now. She loves to run in the morning. She runs all the way to Rehoboth and gets her favorite acai bowl at a local hot spot there and then runs back. She brings a friend and has the time of her life. I love watching her enjoy herself.

Both kids have played piano since they were four. This was Jere's baby. Jere takes piano lessons as well. Me.... I just enjoy watching and listening (most of the time). They started out in the Suzuki method, and then Jere's teacher took over the children's education. We've been lucky to have her. Right around Dell's Bar-mitzvah, the children qualified for the Piano Extravaganza at the forum in Harrisburg. It was a big deal. You had to audition. There were sixteen pianos on stage with two students sitting per each piano at the same time, all playing the same song at the same time led by a conductor. One person plays the top and the other plays the bottom, and every single person and piano must be in rhythm. It's quite challenging. Well, Dell and Bella being two peas in a pod wanted to play together. The only problem with that was there were ten different age categories and ten different levels of strengths or abilities, and Dell was at a much higher level than Bella was. My Bella was determined. She worked and worked, and she and Dell set it up at home. When they tried out, Bella was questioned about her age and if she was prepared to play at this high level. She just sat on the piano bench with her brother and ignored the question. They weren't perfect that day, but it was just a tryout; they were a damn site better than most. When the tiny girl with flaming red hair got down from the piano bench, the instructor just looked at her as she walked away a bit speechless. That was Bella.

Towards the end of middle school, Dell was really having some trouble. Our school district was a mess, the school board was fighting, the teachers were leaving, and there were many disciplinary problems at the school. Dell was in the eighth grade about to embark into high school the following year. It just so happens, Jere and I were discussing what to do about it, when Dell approached us. Now in eighth grade at fourteen, Dell was skinny—maybe four feet and maybe eighty-ninety pounds soaking wet. Dell said," If I keep going to this school, I'm going to turn into a bad kid. I want to go to another school." Wow, this kid is so smart. He was so brave to come to us and see that his future is dire, and he wants a better life for himself at fourteen. Wow, what a remarkable young man. I have never been prouder. I have always believed in listening to your kids and especially now. So we said we don't have a lot of other choices here in Harrisburg, and we can't afford boarding school. There are two excellent Catholic schools to choose from, so Dell shadowed at both, and we let him choose although we secretly had a favorite. He chose our first choice. I was surprised because it was smaller and further away. I asked why he made that choice, and he said that when he went to the other school, he saw too many of the bad kids he knew from his school, and he just wanted a fresh start even if he had to start at a place where he didn't know a single soul.

When Dell Started Trinity High School, it was a huge change for him. He knew nothing but Hebrew School all his life, and he was the sole Jewish kid in the whole school. That can be overwhelming in itself. Part of the mandatory curriculum at the school was everyone must take religious class (Catholic religious class), and everyone had to go to mass every Wednesday. All the kids wore uniforms, and the boys had to shave regularly even if like Dell there wasn't a hair to be seen. He was definitely struggling in religious class but was making his way in the other classes and with the kids. Also, he tried out and made a spot on the soccer team which was a big deal at the school. Then he saw a sign that there was to be an upcoming rap competition in the cafeteria that coming Friday. It didn't give him a lot of time to prepare, but he signed up and started writing. Since his hip hop lessons along with his years of music lessons, Dell had started to become interested in rapping as he called it.

Jere and I weren't sure what to label it at first, but then his writing started to come together. Dell has a natural ear and rhythm. The combination was interesting. The day of the competition had arrived. I honestly didn't realize at the time how huge a deal it was. The whole school, including the faculty, was in the gym. The judges were made up of both students and teachers. It was set up a bit like a gladiator event. The rappers and challengers were in the center, and the peers surrounded them. Several kids went before Dell as was explained to me. They were in crazy costumes and all sorts of things. When it was Dell's turn, he entered not knowing he was allowed to do any of that, so he was in his little skinny school uniform with his little skinny self. He was one of the only freshmen that even signed up. Upperclassmen always win. He goes right up to that microphone, lowers it, of course, and explains loudly and proudly.... "Just so you know, I'm Jewish, and you might not understand some of the words, but they are Jewish words" and proceeds to rap about yarmulke and all sorts of Jewish culture.

Then in the round where they must go toe-to-toe, he holds his own. Long story short he was terrific, and everyone else thought so as well. That day, not only did he end up winning the whole thing, but he also placed himself as a hero in his freshman class for the rest of his time at the school. It was so thrilling that a freshman beat an upperclassman that the valedictorian talked about it in her commencement speech at their graduation. Oh yea, I'd say that was a good day for Dell.

Today Dell is about to start his third year at the University of New Haven majoring in Music Production and Audio Engineering. He is never far from his recording equipment. He makes the most unbelievable music. He is the most sought out producer on campus. It's that ear of his. Look for him at the Grammys, I'll be the proud mom sitting right next to him crying my eyes out. I gave you an indication of my flame-haired lioness Bella, as I like to think of her, and the type of personality she has. She wanted to do everything her brother did—just better. That worked for her for quite some time until she branched off to seek her own fortune. She hip hop danced for years and was quite good. Mom and I would take her once a year to a professional weekend where she had an opportunity to dance with professional choreographers. Mom and I loved watching. It was fabulous. We just couldn't understand how she could pick up those steps so quickly. She also played soccer and had many opportunities. Jere and I went on all the weekend tournaments with her as well hotel to hotel.

Yikes, between the two kids we could have really done a lot of first-class trips with all that money for lessons and hotels for tournaments and soccer dues, but, of course, we wouldn't trade a penny. I did have a few mishaps along the way. Ambulances were called and so forth. It wasn't always bliss, but whatever I could drag myself to I sure did even if I had to rest or whatever it took. This is what I was fighting so hard for, and I was loving every minute.

Bella and Dell both joined BBYO or B'nai Brith Youth Organization, but for Bella she really wanted to follow her mother's footsteps, I think. I was very active as a teenager, and her actions and enjoyment made me so happy. For me, growing up in such a small town, BBYO was my everything. Isabella was a beautiful Bat-Mitzvah. Together she picked her colors to be bright pink and orange. It was so full of life. So did an unbelievable hip- hop contemporary dance. We hired all these back up dancers for her. It was very cool. We had to try and outdo our gold lame', so we came out in disco outfits with huge red wigs for Bella; we messed up the performance thoroughly. YIKES.

The party was fun, and we had a great time. On the bimah after Bella was done with her service, I presented her with my butterfly ring I was given by my grandparents at my Bat-Mitzvah. The ring had meant so much to me as my thirteen-year-old self and now as a mother I was gifting it to my thirteen-year-old daughter hopefully to carry on the tradition to her daughter one day. It was in perfect condition. Bella was thrilled to get it.

Bella decided she wanted to go to Trinity High school as well—what a surprise. It was a fabulous school, and they were kind to us; we wanted her to go there as well. She loved it immediately and did so well right away. She made varsity soccer her first year. She was doing quite well, and she didn't have to take the bus because she had an older brother with a car that just so happened to be going in the same direction. Bella thrived at Trinity making lots of friends and enjoying all the after activities. She had lots of sleepovers. I loved when she had the sleepovers at our house. All the giggling girls were music to my ears. Oh, such fun. Because most of the girls lived further away, she wanted to go to their homes more and I understood, but I had an ace up my sleeve. Most of the parents limited the sleepovers to one person—maybe two—and who could blame them, but I could care less how many girls would sleepover.

By then Dell was in college; she had the whole place. They could lie all over the family room or wherever; it didn't matter to me. I just liked having the girls in the house. I bought pizzas or whatever they wanted—made her favorite chocolate cake and bought the best junk food and always got up in the morning and went out and got her favorite donuts in the morning. I did enjoy the giggling, but as she got a bit older, she didn't want me around so much anymore. No amount of bribery worked. I was just not cool enough anymore. I guess that's just the natural order of things, but I don't have to like it.

We still do lots of other fun girl things. Bella has learned to trust for the most part my sense of fashion. I happen to love fashion. I'm usually quite good at eyeballing the kids or others and choosing the correct size for them when they are not present, and I usually choose things that Bella and even Dell like. But it's even more fun to go shopping together. My mother and I always did that, and we had a ball. I applied the same rule, in fact, that my mom used with me. When Bella found something, we both had to agree on it for her to buy it and same if I found something for her. It made it easy to eliminate any arguments. We picked out beautiful dresses for her dances. That was a new one for me. Dell never wanted to go to the dances. It was such fun. We would get her hair done, and then we would meet up with her friends. I would take pictures of all her friends and all the dates. It was fun. It still is. As I write this book, Bella is just completing her junior year and will begin her senior next year. We are looking into colleges. She is a very bright girl with something like a 4.2 average, and she takes all AP and Honors classes. She works very hard. Every time I see her, she's studying. She's consumed by it. She wants to get into a good business school. They will be lucky to have her. She also works at Starbucks. She looks so cute in her hat. I told her she needs to start saving for college. Dell worked and he saved. He uses a lot of his extra money on his savings.

Ultimately depending on what type of business Bella decides to study, she could end up after her 4 years pursuing an NBA or Law School. However, it's always been her dream to go to Warton, so we will see, but whatever she chooses, she will be a success at it. I know it.

My children approached me that I was spending too much time writing my blog and not enough time with them. I was horrified. I immediately stopped writing, I stopped everything, when I realized what I fought so hard to live for was right in front of me, and my writing was taking up too much time away from them. It was such a wake-up call. I enjoyed writing my blog and connecting with people, but I moved heaven and earth to raise those children, and I wasn't ever going to put that before my children's happiness. As I write about their many accomplishments (and these are just the tip of their many), I realize I definitely made the right choice. We need to be present in our children's lives. The benefits to them benefited me maybe more. My children taught me love, patience, understanding, beauty, laughter, and countless other things. I'm at peace today because I was given the opportunity to meet these amazing human beings. I'm humbled beyond words.

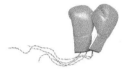

Infection

When I came back from Indiana, it seemed as if I was gone forever. When I walked in the back yard, a few of my friends, were waiting for me which was very sweet. By this time, my tunnel vision was lowering its walls a bit, and I had made it through all three phases of treatment at this point. Not that I didn't think anything couldn't still happen, I was always worried I wouldn't get my treatments, and now that I had gotten them did give me some relief. However, in the back of my mind I always know there is a chance that the insurance companies or my doctors will say there is no longer a need for my medication. Afterall, there is no data for someone like me.

Remember, I am the only one with my aggressive form of cancer, so they have no reason to keep me on my regimen if I am doing well. But I know that one year I had that mammogram, and I was clean and the following year, it was EVERYWHERE.

If I go off this medication, it will be too late to go back on and reverse the outcome. This cancer is far too aggressive. I will worry for the rest of my life.

Anyway, enough of my fun life. Let's get back to the moment at hand, my friends were so surprised to see my Navy men's spiky hair. I hated it; I don't know why, but they all complimented it. I'm not sure I believed them. But it was nice spending time with them. There's no place like home!

I think everyone was happy to be back home. The family was genuinely happy while in Indiana, but now that they were all home; reality set in for them. This was demonstrated for Jere by having to go back to work with all its glorious complications. The children went back to school and got wrapped up in their school activities and sports. Everyone seemed to have their normal to go back to, except me; I had to find my new normal. I wondered what that would look like? I wasn't liking what I was conjuring up, so I didn't.

A good conjure never lasts. My new life came marching on in anyway. The burns are still bad from my radiation. Dr. J. gave me some very good prescription cream that did help, but I am very blistered and the burning in my chest is painful. Now to add insult to injury, I had to go back to chemo. It's not as if I had ever stopped. I went while I was in Indiana. But somehow coming home after all these months and going back to where it all started brought back night terrors ... Green velour blankets, I.V. Poles ... Need I say more—none the less I returned for my maintenance chemo.

Going back wasn't so terrible. Everyone was happy to see me and wanted to know how my radiation treatment had gone and all the details. They were all very kind. They really were the best group of nurses in the business. I was lucky I landed there with them. Soon I was to meet with Dr. M. again. Remember her? She was the doctor during the mastectomy surgery that placed my expanders (Yes, folks she was the good memory during that hell surgery, the one bright light, so let's not confuse her with the other riff raff). Dr. M. was wonderful, so easy going and different than most other plastic surgeons that I know. First, she explained we had to fill back up my expanders and wait several months to see if we could expand my skin.

I don't think I lasted with those things for two weeks before I landed myself in the hospital. I was feeling really bad and crappy—not sure what was going on. I just endured, but things went from bad to worse fast. I just felt worse and worse, and my temperature started to spike, so I contacted the doctor when I couldn't stand it any longer. I was urged to hightail it to Johns Hopkins. It seems that I had gotten an infection from the expanders. Who knew that could happen?? Only me.

Of course, I'm the poster child for disaster of the worse kind. I remember something I was told once in a kind way, but the impact was the same; I always seemed to get the worst case of poison ivy or worse case of food poisoning; however small or simple, mine would always be the worst or so I was told; it just was (and it's seeming in all things cancer, I'm not only living up to that reputation but excelling at it). This particular infection really sucked. I was horribly nauseous and had a temperature. They had to rush me into surgery if you can believe it, SURGERY for crying out loud, and flush out my whole chest so I didn't die .... hahahaha Isn't that funny. "Woman struggles desperately to survive metastatic cancer only to die horribly from infection from breast expanders. News at ten."

Fortunately, I stayed off the ten o'clock news but barely. I was in the hospital for over a week. After the surgery, they left these drains hanging outside of my body, and they were still in when I went home. There was a lot to drain apparently. I could hardly look; it was so gross. You could see all this blood and guts coming out of my body. It was connected by a tube running inside me, so if I was sleeping, it would pull, and it would burn like hellfire, I mean really. It was truly horrible. I hated those damn things!!!! They hurt like hell. They would hang from me and swing around. I would get those things you wear around your neck with a whistle and attach it to each drain somehow. Let's say I had four drains. Then I'd have four necklaces around my neck. It sounds crazy, but it took the pressure off the wound site and helped. (I believe they are called lanyards.) I still find them all over the house now; they just represent so much more to me than their innocent appearance suggests. They give me the heebeegeebees when I see them, even though I thought it was a very inventive use of my children's soccer materials. It was quite a while before they were finally done draining and were removed.

YAY! Meantime, I must heal, but Dr. M. and I discussed what we do next. There are not really a lot of reconstruction options for me. There is no option for implants. First of all, I pretty much just proved that with having this last infection so quickly. There had been so much damage done to my chest wall that she had already told me I wouldn't be a candidate for implants.Therefore, I was left with a trans flap. A trans flap is basically where you take some of your own viable tissue from somewhere that works compatibility with breast tissue and transfer it onto the breast along with fat. Now if Dr. M. could have taken it from my ass, she could have given me the hugest bazingas ever. That's ok ... I definitely didn't want huge bazingas. I had 'em—didn't wanted me back!!!! Just making a point. You all get the picture .... big ass, right? You with me so far? So that was my end game, but a lot had to happen for me to get there. Dr. M. said. " We should try to fill the expanders again. We don't know if that was a fluke, and there's no reason to think it should happen again. I really need your tissue to expand." (The whole time right after surgery—meaning my mastectomy—when it was the most important, I was in Indiana and was not expanded. That was a crucial time.) "so, if this is what you want, we should really try again."

I said "Okay", but I was conjuring a plane crashing down and a terrorist killing us all in a fiery death of flames. I stared them in the face and said with gusto, "Let's roll." I can be a bit dramatic at times I am told. Don't believe a word of it. Back to where us undramatic people were ... So, we expanded the expanders AGAIN.

FUN! FUN! FUN! I mean it's a party at my house wa-hooooo. Boobees again. If you could call them that.

Weird—they are just weird. Have you ever seen an expander? They are weird. Did I mention they are weird? I have square lopsided weird boobs, and they hurt. Yeah, they hurt!!

I press on because that's what I do. That's me alright. The presser owner. And guess what happened? No, I mean you have to guess ... Really??? Have you guessed yet? Hmmm? Ok I'll tell you and put you out of your misery (and it better be misery) I Got Another Infection and Ended Back in the Hospital!!! Oh Yes, I Did!!!@!! It took longer the second time, but the result was the same—back at Johns Hopkins in the hospital having to get the same surgery. This time was not quite as smooth; not that hospital visits are smooth. It's just that they didn't have a room available on the cancer floor for me, so I had to wait in this holding area, and I was getting sicker and more uncomfortable. Then they tried to access my arm to give me some fluids and take blood, but I am a very hard stick because of chemo treatments. Remember, I am only able to use one arm—my poor sad arm. Needless to say, this arm by now wasn't doing very well, and needed one of those special stick nurses which I tried to tell them, but OH NO, everyone thinks they are the very best at their trade, and I am sure that at most times they are but not on my poor one arm that was sorely dehydrated. It ensued from there, and stick became stick until I vomited all over them.

Then they called in the big guns. However, they still needed to access me between my toes that day. Let me tell you, that was unpleasant. Meanwhile, my poor mother was by my side through it all. Yikes, reviewing it all backwards. I think she had the short end of the stick. Jere arrived and shouldered some of her worry as I was led to my room. Finally, we saw Dr. M., and she said "yep" another surgery, and I would need the same drains put in burning and dangling from me. Just great, huh?? After surgery I typically get nauseous, and we all know by now how much I love blood tests. Now, while I'm in my room, very, very nauseated, I hear a chipper voice. I slowly and I mean slowly look up; I see a girl my daughter's age come in with what I call the" coke bottle" because that's what it's shaped like—an old-fashioned regular Coca Cola bottle—coming toward me. She says, "It's time to get your blood culture." (What the hell does that mean?) "We need to test your blood for all types of infections to find out which infection you have in case it's dangerous for you or something."

"Oh shit, come on now. Puh- Lease give me a break. You mean you are going to take all that blood from my body? I can't take any more. I'm telling you." As she takes my blood, I begin to get very nauseous and start to go down and down ... oh my, there she blows. Then nothing. Well, I don't remember any smile on her fucken chipper face now. Huh??? Told ya!!! They still try every time I'm in a hospital to bring me that coke bottle. It doesn't matter who that fucking chipper smile belongs to, I kick them out of my room so fast they don't have time to pick that smile up off that floor in time before I wipe it up with my hospital socked foot.

I can still see some of those grill marks on some of the girls that weren't quick enough. No more coke bottles for me!!! Yes, I regress with my childishness. I ended up with yet a second infection and was hospitalized for again about a week and came home with the dreaded drains. I had quite a few in this time, and Dr. M. felt as if they should stay in extra- long just to make sure all the infection was clear. I thought maybe it was just to torture me for torturing the nurse that tried to administer the coke bottle. Just kidding. I was nice to all the floor nurses; the coke bottle nurse came from a different floor. Ha tricked ya. This was a longer recovery. Each one was tougher on my body, and each one was more difficult for me to recover from. Also, we mustn't forget I'm still getting chemo treatment through all of this mess. I think my oncologist made me miss one appointment because my numbers were so low (they take blood and so forth before they even order your medication), and I wasn't doing well and was green when I turned up for treatment, but even so I turned up. No matter what, I will always be there.

Nothing is more important to me ... NOTHING. I was not happy that I couldn't get my chemo that day. Not Happy. After all I had driven two hours in pain to get there; the least I could have been given was more pain Thank You very much. I rest my case.

Unfortunately, since yes, I was weaker this time, and Dr. M. had decided to keep my drains in longer, all of it crescendo up against The Book Fair I have overseen since my son was in the first grade, a long time ago because at this point, I'm at a different school. Anyway, I'm weak. It's a huge undertaking, and I've got these scary bloody drains hanging from me, which is perfect for third, fourth, and fifth graders to see, don't you think? They need education, too, right? Oh, my goodness, but I had just about the best partner. We had been doing the Book Fair together since the beginning, and we worked together terrific. Most book fairs before ours weren't half as organized or well run because we were sort of yin and yang and also because we genuinely liked each other and worked so well together. I think it showed. I attended (oh come, on you knew I would). However, I did cut some hours back and didn't do any heavy lifting. Again, thank goodness for such a strong partner. It's a lot of work. But I wore a big jacket to hide my drains, and we were off and selling. It was fun. I used to love those Book Fairs. A friend of mine told me Scholastic rearranged all the original staff during COVID and ruined the flavor of the company. I thought it used to be about reading and schools. They could have helped those poor teachers struggling and parents during such a tough time which is what my friend and all her original staff members wanted, but they brought in young flashy people that didn't understand teachers. How ironic. But again, I digress. Sorry. I was happy to be able to participate with one of my pet projects. I was President of the PTO just maybe over a year or two prior to this Fair. Wow, it's amazing how things can change on a dime. I love being active in my kids' school and their lives. I was thankful to my friend for giving me the opportunity to be there and be useful and help.

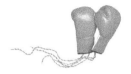

The Bar-Mitzvah

In the ensuing months Dr. M. wanted me to take my time to heal before we pressed on with a decision, so I waited and healed. I refuse to give up just because my body chooses to. The expanders are very uncomfortable, but I will put up with anything to keep my dream of having some semblance of a bod back. You must understand, when I stand, in front, of the mirror, it's so completely strange. I refer to myself as a eunuch. I feel as if that's kind of what I look a bit like ... scars everywhere, like something out of a roadmap ... but to nowhere and nowhere good—that's for sure. Then there's the boob situation, and that's all a bit of a mess. I'm flat and scarred; then I get expanded again, slowly mind you, so lump by lumpy - lump ... until, I'm all square and weird. Then it begins all over again in the hospital where I deflate, and the bloody drains go hanging from me like something out of a Dracula film, and so on and so on. Are you kind of getting the picture now??

Instead of wasting time staring at myself in the mirror, I decided just to enjoy finishing planning my beautiful son's Bar-Mitzvah. After all, didn't someone say I wouldn't make it to this big day? Didn't I have a lot to celebrate? Hell, Ya, I did!! So, let's get to it. There was so much hope and blood and sweat and tears and hope and fear placed onto this Bar-Mitzvah, that I just didn't know what I thought as the months rolled around and the invitations started coming in. Like HOLY FUCKIN SHIT. THIS THING MIGHT REALLY COME OFF. But then more quietly I say to myself—oh my, why did you just say that???? OH, OH, OH, quick jazz hands. That's my version of trying to tell myself to shut up. (Jazz hands make me puke.)

Sorry, I regress when I begin to speak to myself in my own book. That's how I know and you now just how completely crazy I am, Folks. I'm just getting nervous for the "ME", back then, all over again. It's horrible how tough this time was for us all. But it was also a groundbreaking,

FUCKING AWESOME time as well. You wonder, how the worst time can be our best time, and all I can say is decide for yourself. It was a busy time for me. I was very weak still from all the recent infections. I had barely healed but was happy and planning every last detail. However, would you believe? Of course, you would, because who am I asking at this point—what a ridiculous question. What I'm asking you to "believe" is yet another roadblock in my constant upsets in my journey. Yet again I was being challenged, and in comes my constant upper respiratory infection after infection— one after another. Practically living on antibiotics which weren't good for me or my immune system, so they (the powers that be) decided to have my tonsils removed at the last minute. Can you believe that??? I sure as hell couldn't believe it. No one thought I would make it to the Bar-Mitzvah for sure now. Nobody believed I would be able to recover in time. Well, for all you suckers, I'm like the Little Engine That Could. Did you ever read that book as a child? I think I can, I think I can, I think I can, I think I can, I think I can ... .

That's me choo choo' chooing along. And I CAN!!! CUZ NO ONE TELLS ME I CAN'T!!

God Bless my friends—again to the rescue!! All of those invitations that came in that I was so tickled about—that I described earlier—my most wonderful and amazing friends all came over to my house, grabbed my list when I couldn't, and got into what could only be described as a bucket brigade a sort of set up around my kitchen table handing everything off like professional ball players, and as you can see, all the invites made their way to the proper person, even Israel. They are pretty fanfuckintastic, my friends!!! How about that, right!!! I must have done something right along the way. I'm just baffled by what it must have been.

Getting back to the party stuff and planning the BM (I'M going to call the Bar-Mitzvah from here on out the BM—yes, get a good old laugh out now. Ha Ha- funny funny. Ok, are you all ready to quit your potty jokes and stop laughing whenever I say BM. Ready???)

Planning the BM took a lot of work and effort, but it was as if I was made for this. I have been praying for this for so long;

I was enjoying every minute of it. Remember, earlier in my "story" I had been telling you about when I was told by Dr. E., a doctor that I had trusted and developed a relationship with and who had told me I would not be alive for my son's Bar-Mitzvah? If you don't remember, I sure as hell do; any how this venue is the location I marched all "sassy like" down to their office with a check in hand (maybe shaking just a bit) and put down a deposit on the room in which we will have our beautiful reception after the service.

How about that, Folks? Let's just soak that in for a moment.... Hmmmmm, WOW! HOLY COW SHIT! RIGHT How surreal is that? It goes to show you there's a lot to be said for blind faith. i. e. this is a lucky place. We are going to have a great party here; I can feel it! The ironic thing is it was getting a bit pricier than we had budgeted because we had underestimated the number of "no's" we would get in response to our invitation. Yep, that's right, Folks, the dreaded, we didn't get any. Yes, we loved everyone we invited. BUT NOBODY AND I MEAN NOBODY INVITES EVERYONE THINKING EVERYONE IS GOING TO SHOW UP!! I mean really people, haven't you ever planned a party and were down to your last buck and you were ready to charge for the door that showed up and responded "yes"? You know you thought it, so you might as well fess up. That's just about where we were, but we were so happy we just didn't care—medical bills and all. This was just too much of a joyous occasion, and we were just too damn grateful.

I was determined to give everyone a good show.

The kids set out to rehearse a piano performance to perform during the party. The venue had a beautiful piano, and they said would they bring it into the main room for us to use which was fantastic. As the kids practiced their piano, Jere and I practiced our dance. Oh yes, you heard me correctly. When I say put on a show, I mean you come to a party where I come back from the dead and my son becomes a BAR-MITZVAH and you will get a show!!! HELL TO THE YA!

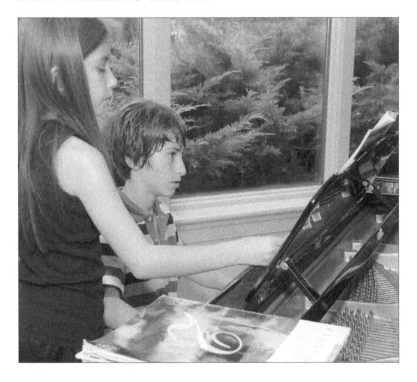

We hired my son's hip-hop teacher because as I mentioned, he was going to do a break dance, and we were going to be his surprise guest back up dancers, including Isabella who could learn her steps in five minutes. It took her father and me a bit longer....

There are so many little details involved—like the program and who goes up to be honored. We have a strict procedure at our Temple that I needed to adhere too, and I can only select a certain number and must keep to the rules. I have so many personalities; it's tough to choose. I want everyone to stand up on the bimah to stand with my son before God and wish him well as he becomes a man. We all love him, and everyone has waited for this day to come if only I could just choose everyone. I wonder if my cousins who are going through their own Bar- and Bat-Mitzvahs now are having as much difficulty with this problem as I did then.

The big day had finally arrived. How exciting. All the pretty clothes we bought were all hanging and ready to go. I probably should have mentioned this is a huge production if you have not figured that out yet. A Bar-Mitzvah is like a wedding. This is a whole weekend event—oh yes, event because I have the whole weekend planned. All our out-of-town friends and family members are pouring into sleepy Harrisburg by airplane, by car, and by train, and all are headed to their hotel or friends' homes. Everyone is enjoying the welcome bags that I personally prepared with my lovely friends—bags all with my son's Bar-Mitzvah colors of blue and silver; bags with his name on them and lots of goodies inside. Everyone is happy to see one another or is taking a nap while waiting for the festivities to begin.

Everyone piled into the chapel at the synagogue Friday night in early November. It sure was chilly already. I'm not sure the last time this chapel saw so many people. It wasn't prepared for my crew—that's for sure—because we were pulling chairs from everywhere to manage everyone. It was kind of cozy though— all of us squeezed together for the beginning of our weekend together. It was the first time I was seeing most everyone, so we were waving joyously across the room. The service was a family affair. Dell went up and did his thing. I went up and lit the candles. Bella went up and did the closing song with her brother. It was fun. After the service, we headed to the Country Club; my kind and generous mother was hosting the evening dinner. It was lovely. Everyone had an opportunity to finally let off steam and talk freely and catch up.

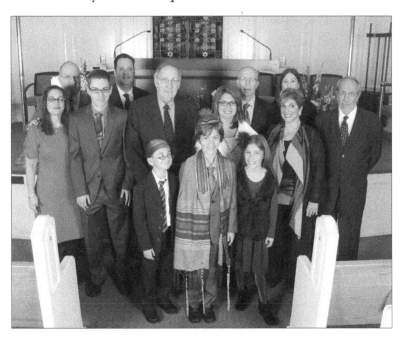

The big day has arrived, and I'm not quite sure who is more nervous at this point. Anybody could point to any of us at any given time, and we would jump out of our skin as if it was on fire. Our immediate family got up at the crack of dawn, so we could get some family photos at the synagogue before everyone arrived. That nasty chill was back in the air, and it was tough taking our coats off for those perfect outdoor photos that showed off our pretty outfits. But anything for a photo op. The rest of our family and friends that we didn't see Friday night, we now got an opportunity to see. Everyone looked so pretty, all dressed up in all their bright colors.

The synagogue never looked better. However, on a side note, it almost didn't because I forgot to order the flowers for the synagogue, and last night's chapel. If the Temple hadn't called me and said they would just order them with my permission and bill me, I would have been S.O.L. I was very happy they called me. The flowers I paid for were quite lovely, if I must say so myself.

The Temple seemed to be buzzing with anticipation. Even Dell started to get a bit overwhelmed and needed a minute. We hurried him into a back room along with our friend, The Rabbi Peter. "Ok, Dell, what's going on," I asked. "Are you ready for this? Because I know of a back way out where no one will be able to see us leave. What do you think? Do you want to hightail it out of here? Or since maybe you did study for two years to get to this day; and there is a really cool party at the end, would you like to just finish it?" (He's thinking....)

"I guess I might as well finish. If you are going to do this, do it well. Remember we talked about no mumbling, head up, speak so everyone can understand, pause, and so forth. I got this, Mom."

"I never doubted it, Dell. We'll be right there with you."

The Rabbi came out, and most of the service was a blur to me. I remember a couple of things. I remember that Dell did do all those things that I asked him to do and then some. He really was terrific. He spoke well with confidence and gave pause for laughter; he really did a nice job. I was proud of him. Tears did slide down my cheeks, but it was that kind of day.

When it came time for the honors, my family members came up to the bimah in two's like from Noah's ark and said their prayer, went around the table, kissed Dell and left; this continued until the last honor which was ours; by now something like relief was taking over and great nerves for what lie ahead, so I just got the giggles at this poorly timed moment. I muddled through the prayer with a snort and a giggle and a smile, went around the table, and kissed my son.

When the service was complete, Jere and I went up and spoke about how proud we were of Dell and all his accomplishments. I love the young man he is turning out to be—the young man who had the strength of character to come to us and say if I stay in this school, I`m afraid I might turn into a bad kid. That takes guts. This boy is now a man who is going to do good things in this World. I just hope I'm around to see it because it's really going to be something. Jere spoke a bit, and a couple of other gifts were given out. Our sweet little Bella came forward to sing the last song with Dell, and the ceremony was over just like that.

So many things were flashing into my head at that very moment. It was as if I had a whoosh go by me like a flash before my eyes. Was this a warning, showing me how lucky I am and not to squander it? Was it just showing my life pass before my eyes because GOD was going to take me now? I didn't believe that one; or was it a gentle reminder of my promise to God. Either way I knew I would keep that promise, and if this was it, I wanted to enjoy my family and friends and soak every single moment in. I made sure all the children had rides to our reception, and I sat quietly for just a minute on the bimah appreciating the day and closing my eyes to burn it into my memory. "I made it," I said quietly to myself, and an arm shot in the air like a rocket ready for take-off. I embraced the moment alone as tears streamed down my face. "I made it," I said softly again.

By the time we got to the venue, the DJ Adam Weitz from Philadelphia was already done setting up, and the dancers were out on the floor; the party was a REAL party! Everything looked so lovely; I just couldn't believe I had painstakingly picked everything out myself. As I learned from my mother, I gave myself a big "Atta Boy" on the shoulder and a little twirl admiring all my hard work napkin by napkin, plate by plate. It was a site to behold, and excitement and a giggle bubbled up inside me. Man, oh man when I got it, I got it. Now, Girl, let's go show 'em what else you got. And off I went....

The party started off with a cocktail hour (it's really longer than an hour) with hor d'oeuvres for the adults on one side of the room (at our affair I wanted us to all be in the same room, but each doing our own thing. Most often the kids are in one room—the adults in another). Adam, our DJ, was really entertaining the kids. Every time I glanced over to see if Dell was enjoying his party, he was having a blast. The DJ had professional dancers with him; they were playing games with the kids. Dell and Bella had teamed up together much to the dismay of his friends who all wanted to team up with him. But both Dell and Isabella were very competitive and knew that not only could they count on each other, but even though Bella was three years younger, she was still the second fastest person in the whole room—only second to her brother. She definitely didn't disappoint, because before I turned away, I saw them win the game that they were playing. This was the reason I kept us all in the same room. I could see the huge smiles on my children's faces, that I witnessed at that very moment. It is and always will be burned into my memory. Who wouldn't want that for a memory?

I must say the kids' side of the room did look way more fun than the grownup side. We had nice conversation and fancy food and booze, but the kids' side had games with good looking dancers and greasy yummy food. There was candy at every table and a huge table where anyone could dress in silly hats or glasses and take pictures with friends and pick out a cool frame to keep so they can remember the party. Prizes were being thrown out onto the dance floor. The best part was when I looked over and saw our young cousins up on the stage dancing and whipping to the Nae Nae song.

(OMG, you can't even imagine how cute these kids were, shaking it up on that stage.) The grownups were having a great time as well. Some of us don't get to see each other very often, so there was a lot of catching up and showing off pictures in our wallets. The photographer was wandering around taking pictures of myself with all my besties and family candid's. Other people that didn't know too many people were getting to know everyone and exchanging numbers to keep in touch. It was quite nice to step back, and just take it all in. The invited group was a nice mix of people, and everyone seemed so happy just to be there that day.

While I was taking stock in my head, we were all called to the table for our first course, and that was my cue for the beginning of our surprise. We sat along with everyone for a minute and then covertly slipped away. First Adam, (remember the DJ) played a prearranged song to announce each member of our family as we were formally brought out and introduced to our guests. Jere and I were called first, and people were lined up on either side. We came up the middle hand in hand dancing and twirling to "The Fight Song"; it had just come out and made quite the impact when it was played. Then little Bella came out Cleopatra style held up high like the princess that she is. I think it was a Taylor Swift Song. Then our big guy, the star of the night, Dell, walked out all cool struts flanked by dancers throwing around monopoly money to some rap song about money. So cute but don't tell him I said that. From there my uncle, aunt, and I believe his two daughters did the prayer for the bread and wine.

Then everyone was seated at their reserved tables, and the salads were served. While everyone was eating their salads, the kids, Jere, and I slipped out to our secret spot to change into our costumes to await our cue. When everyone had finished their salads, they were asked to get up and stand around the dance floor; they were in for a real treat. The music started, and boy, did Dell blow right onto that stage. He flew right out and slid right on his knees all hip- hop style and proceeded to go from trick to trick. He was very good, very rhythmic, very impressive. Everyone kept clapping. We had his music mixed by his hip hop teacher, so when the "You Can't Touch This" song by M. C. Hammer (oh yeah, it's Hammer Time) came on, that was our cue to enter the stage. The crazy thing is I left a part out that you need to know, so you can fully comprehend what everyone was witnessing. I had purchased gold lame' costumes for Jere, Isabella, and me. They consisted of gold lame' vests and huge gold lame' pants with a really low hung crotch as Hammer al-ways used to wear, and we all wore black shiny shoes.

Well, if you can imagine, we barely hit the floor before tears of laughter were running down people's faces. They never had seen anything like it. They couldn't believe we had the balls to look that ridiculous in front of everyone and then dance hor-ribly. No one knew what to laugh at the most, the dancing or the costumes. We only had a three-minute set before Dell came back on, but people still talk about that today. It was worth all the hard work of trying to find costumes for each of our sizes and learning the dance when I had a major chemo brain and two left feet.

Seeing everyone have such a good time was worth it. I also wanted to demonstrate to my children that fear should never hold them back from the things they want to do in life. Leaning into whatever your fear may be hard; embarrassment is always a big one, but never allow embarrassment to take your power away. Lean into it kids. It will work itself out. A little embarrassment can't hurt you. Take its power by having fun! And that's what we did; we had fun. I still have those costumes today because if my kids ever need that lesson, I'll just have them put on that costume and wear it to school with a sign on its back that says, "You Can't Touch This".

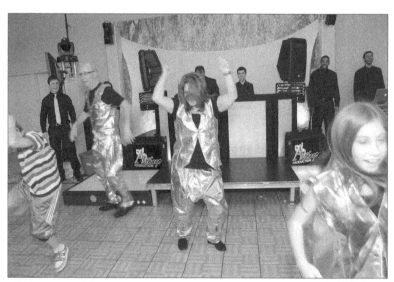

After the dance everything was pandemonium. Everyone came running over to us and Dell. They didn't know Dell could dance so well. Where did he learn to do that? and on and on.... Then to us—where did we get our costumes? How did we come up with our dance steps? What balls we had. How everyone loved it.... It was nice and fun. I'm glad we did it. Now I was wondering why we were not being seated for our main course, so I snuck away in search of my contact to find out why. Well, it turns out that they blew a fuse and were distracted, not sure why and didn't realize that the ovens had turned off some time ago, and nothing was cooked. Needless to say, our meal was far from ready. Everyone was going to get restless if we didn't do something quickly, so I suggested to our DJ that we change up the schedule a bit, so we could dance some. I would go change clothes; then he would call me to the microphone for my speech. I would just give it early. I, of course, had filled him in.

I was pretty tired at this point; my body had been through quite a bit to get to this day, so I really wanted to rest but was fearful to do that in case the party would get out of hand because everyone would get anxious about dinner. I changed as quickly as I could, and off I went. People could see that I was pale and stopped me along the way to sit down or have something to drink. It was a bit longer than I expected until I got to the DJ, but he was clearly a professional and had things well at hand. I should have never worried. He had children and adults alike doing all sorts of things along with his dancers. It was really funny.

I almost turned around to go sit down in a peaceful spot, but damn it's too late—he spotted me and signaled me to come over to his side. He introduced me and handed me the microphone. I just looked at it for a second exhausted; then the second wave took hold, and I began. I am not sure I remember much of what I said ... bits and pieces. But this was a very different speech than the one I spoke from that morning's Bimah at the temple service. Not only was I given a time limit there, but I also felt that, that speech should have one type of content more related to his work and studies and his haftorah portion and thanking his teachers and so forth. This speech was more personal, about our family, and all we have been through to get here to this exact day. I spoke of how I taught Dell elocution lessons for his own speech on the bimah today and how well he did—how proud I was of him and what a wonderful son he is. I spoke of his extracurricular activities, that not only does he dance but he raps as well and plays the piano. Then I spoke of gratitude for my amazing friends and listed the many things they did to assist in getting me to this day in one piece. I spoke a bit of my personal struggle and what it has meant to me to be here on this day when "I was told I wouldn't be standing here, let alone ever getting this opportunity to look out at all my favorite people in the whole world in one room and get to share this most important moment in my life with you all. To get to see the triumph on my son's face when his haftorah portion was over; to see and hear the laughter of everyone when we came out in our ridiculous gold lame' outfits. I may have had cancer through the left side of my heart, but it sure didn't keep it from soaring today." Now we are going to do this all again in three years because I promised a little redhead, my beautiful daughter Isabella; that we would all get to do this all over again for her." (She wants whatever her brother gets but always with a twist). Then I lifted my fist into the air for yeah and Halleluiah. What's interesting here is I was so determined, I knew one hundred percent that I was going to make Isabella's Bat-Mitzvah in three years just as I knew I would make Dell's, but those closest to me that saw my x- rays and knew my prognosis were afraid and rightfully so, but didn't really share this with me until recently, because of this book.

I never knew their misgivings and fears. I was oblivious to it all the stares everyone was exchanging when I made that statement. I was just moving forward. It's good, so I can give you all the other perspectives. This is what's interesting; just as that comment comes out of my mouth, my very best friend who is "my person" literally cringed when I publicly made a promise to my young daughter that I would make her Bat-Mitzvah in three years. In discussing this with her today, she said it really upset her at the time as well as others. Those would be the people that would have to pick up the pieces that I leave behind if I were to lose my battle. I don't say that flippant or with malice, oh my no. I say this because looking at it from her point of view, maybe she was right. Maybe I shouldn't have made such cavalier promises. Yes, I was sure. I felt in my GUT, I was going to make it, and my positive words saying them out loud so much helped me, I believe. How does the saying go … ? Until you say it out loud, it won't come true. I guess it's kind of like putting it out there in the universe. But still I would not have wanted to scare or hurt anyone's feelings. Back then I was still pretty much fight or flight. And I was all FIGHT FIGHT FIGHT. I didn't even acknowledge flight.

Looking back, I'd say there's a lot to say about positive thinking, but it's not only positive thinking you really have to BELIEVE it, and I absolutely did. That's what gave me my edge so to speak, I believed, and I still believe. I believe in myself. I believe in God and my spirituality and a dream I had a very long time ago, long before I even got sick, and I believe what I feel in my instincts. Some think that sounds a bit crazy, and it probably is crazy, but a little bit of crazy is interesting. A little bit of crazy got my here today—ten years later. I wonder where a little bit of crazy will take me next??? Adam had everyone dancing on the dance floor when they finally called us to our tables for dinner. Well, geez Louise, thank goodness. We all sat down to eat, and the food was delicious. At least for me, it was worth the wait, I hope everyone else felt the same. As dinner was winding down, Dell and Bella headed over to the piano, and Adam announced them as the children began to play. They were terrific together. I think everyone was pleasantly surprised. They didn't know what to expect. They were so adorable. Boy, did I luck out in the kid department. They are going to do good things in this lifetime. I am already seeing that prediction come true today. They are twenty-one and eighteen today and terrific humans. After the piano playing, we served dessert. There was a huge ice cream sundae bar, Dell's favorite, and all kinds of other stuff:

lemon bars for my mom, cookies of all kinds, other pastries, too many to count. I don't remember them all, but everyone had a ball tasting a little bit of everything.

Not too much longer after dessert people started getting ready to leave, you could see the exhausted look on their faces. Dinner being held up so long did kind of throw everyone off a bit. But everyone didn't leave before they took a bag and went to the huge candy station I had set up before you walked out the door and scooped up a huge bag of candy to take home with them. All in all, the party was a big success. I looked over for a minute, and I saw the funniest sight of the whole night. Dell was face down in the middle of the dance floor was fast asleep — totally conked out from sheer exhaustion. His hair was soaked from sweat. I never saw anything so adorable in all my life. Even though I got a photo of that moment, I can conjure up that memory photo in my head just as easily.

After paying all the personnel and packing up the cars with the gifts and all of our things we needed to bring back home, we needed to get going because I had to get the house ready for another party, I was hosting at my home in two hours for all of the out-of-town family and friends that were staying in hotels and such.

When I pulled up, the wait staff I had hired was already at work, because my dad went back to the house early for me to let them in so they could get started. Yay, DAD!! They had everything well at hand, and I had set everything up prior. All the rental tables were set up, and the house looked pretty good, so everyone went off to change into yet another outfit. I came out, paid for the food delivery, and was lighting all the candles as people were starting to pour into the house; the latest party was under way. This was nice because it was more intimate, and I wasn't all keyed up with every little detail as I was earlier in the day. Here I could finally relax, sit down with all my favorite cousins, and catch up with them— spend some time with them. I missed them so much and loved them so. They had been so amazingly supportive of me in the last two years, and I worried I didn't show my appreciation (remember tunnel vision, fierceness in my healing kept me so focused). I also wanted to take some time to spend with my Michelle as you know how much I love her. Even that night got away from me. I did spend time with all those people I mentioned, but there were still other's that had come from all over that I needed to personally thank for coming. My time was split, and I sure was exhausted by the time everyone had left. Now I know you are going to think I'm crazy when I say there is still one more gathering to this shindig.

The next morning, depending on planes, trains, and automobiles everyone was invited back over to my place for brunch. The same amazing servers came back, and I had huge platters made up of bagels and fishes and kugels made and fruit, and we had leftover cookies and all kinds of treats. Everyone stayed several hours and talked about the weekend and all the highlights. All in All, it was well worth all the work and expense. It was the greatest weekend of my life. So much anticipation and buildup sometimes lead to let down. Do you know what I mean? Whatever we picture in our heads or our imaginations we can't possibly live up to. How could we? It's not real. It's impossible to live up to a dream of a ghost, but this did. This weekend lived up to it and more. Here it is ten years later, and the thought of that weekend draws great emotion from me. It's not only telling about the significance of this memory (after all the chemical makeup to my brain has significant changes due to long term use of chemotherapy) but of the emotional attachment I have to it that I am constantly recalling it repeatedly and again.

So when the last person left our home and it was just the four of us again and we were all plopped down in the family room together and we just looked at each other too exhausted to speak, I'm thinking how are we going to get up tomorrow morning and go about our day as if it were a regular day and nothing monumental has just happened. Jere has to go to work tomorrow morning. The kids have to get up for school. Who even knows what I have to fake to do tomorrow? It's going to be a tough day.

I suggested to the kids to go and take baths, and there we have it, Folks ... back to normal. "Mom, do we have to? I want to play with my new toys. But mom it's too early to take a bath." ... And when I turned to smile at Jere, he was fast asleep on the couch. Yep, back to normal, alright.

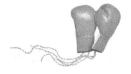

Thank You

I was finally in a place that I felt I could at least thank some of those that were so unbelievably helpful to me outside of my family members; of course, they were in a different stratosphere. I just had such overwhelming gratitude for all of them. If people tell me today that I am a giving person or I am a gracious person, it is because I learned it from this group of people. They taught me kindness to others and giving without the need for a quid pro quo; they wanted nothing in return. They were totally selfless. Those are all lessons I learned from this amazing group of people. I will forever and always be grateful for them and to them. I learned how to treat people in their greatest time of need. How I was given such grace and respect and space and unconditional love is something I will pay forward for the rest of my life. I learned all of that from all of them. I will always be grateful for what I learned from my amazing posse. I love being kind and gracious, and I THANK YOU.

There was no other choice but to throw a party at a restaurant and do a proper Thank You with booze. Everyone had a good time. So many people to thank, but I could only invite so many because the restaurant was only big enough for a certain number; the people that helped the most were there. I was so proud to be able to thank them. I did stand up and properly tell them, and that was a proud moment for me because it was important to me to look everyone in the eye personally and thank them from my heart. I needed them to know I was appreciative because remember my "TUNNEL VISION" period couldn't have been easy for them—not getting any love back from me. That must have been tough for them feeling maybe they were giving and not being appreciated, yet they kept giving. You see that's a sign of a true friend not seeking anything in return, truly just wanting to give; it must have been difficult for them, I would think. I mean I was kind of out there sometimes. I was off somewhere in another world fighting bad guys in my head, certainly not paying any attention to them. I'm just trying to say to everyone involved or anyone reading this that is connecting to these words, hang in there; this is an example of who you want by your side when disaster hits. It was a very nice night. One for the memory book.

I only wish I had done one for my family as well. You know I most certainly have thanked my family members each individually in a heartfelt manner, and I show my appreciation and gratitude to them in many ways, but I think it would have been nice to have dinner for them as well. Maybe it's not too late? When you get this book, you all can check in with my website and tell me what you think. How about that? I do have an absolutely awesome family. I haven't gone into much detail; maybe I should.

You have heard many stories about my mom. Well, if you are ever on a ship and it's sinking, it's my mom that you want to be next to because she will get you home and safe. It's her specialty. As any mother and daughter, we have had our moments, but we have always been able to have an honest conversation and work our way through it. She really is quite remarkable. The best mother a girl could ask for. I definitely hit the mom lottery and am so grateful for her every day. She still drives me to all my chemotherapy treatments. Everyone can't believe it. Some that don't know her look at me with a frown as if I'm an elder abuser or something, and I look back at them and say, "My mom drives better than probably you and better than anyone in my family, she drives like Mario Andretti, and she looks younger than I am and has twice the energy of Sylvester Stallone, so lay off"! That's Mom; she's a firecracker. She is always there for the three of us, my brother and sister included. She is an amazing woman. As far as I am concerned, the sun rises and sets on my mom!!!

You have also heard a bit about my sister or "sistah," as we often refer to each other. We are almost five years apart so when we were younger that was a big deal. She had Mom and Dad all to herself before I came along, and that was unacceptable in her young mind. She would set me up, before I could even speak, and get me in all sorts of trouble, like the time she pushed me into a room we weren't allowed to be in as kids, and picked up a precious vase, put it into my hands, then ran out of the room, and yelled, "MOM, Viki is in the living room with the vase", and, of course, everyone would come running, and I would get into trouble. She loved this but played it one too many times until she was caught, and well, you don't want to know the grisly details of that one. As I got older, I had the opportunity to go to the same summer camp where she was a counselor. That was the best summer of my life because my sister noticed me. I felt so good that she paid attention to me. I thought maybe she even liked me a little. I had always hoped she would. She was so cool and pretty and all of that and had so many friends. We were at that camp for a month, and it was the best month of my childhood hands down! I even have tears—no, actually, I am flat out crying just remembering it and what it meant to that little girl in me. Best month of my life, hands down. That's the summer I got a sister. Unfortunately for me, when we got back, she was preparing to leave for college, so she was off again in only a couple of weeks. That was tough for me. But she didn't forget me, and we were friends ever since our camp days no matter where each of us was. We always keep in close touch. We always talk for hours, and she always has my back. When I got sick, it was very difficult for her. I know she wants to take the pain away for me. To make things tougher for her, she feels removed. She and her family all live in Pittsburg while I live in Harrisburg, and Mom lives right next door just one town over, only about thirty minutes away. My dad is just in Reading, only ninety minutes away, so she feels helpless not being able to participate as much as everyone else. In addition, she's a teacher, so she's limited in the time she can take off. But every time she made it to a chemotherapy session it was fun. She makes everything fun. She's a ray of light wherever she goes, and I find that comforting. My sister is the sister you want in your corner. I lucked out again. Now I've got a great mom and a cool and compassionate sister. How lucky am I? I told you all I hit the family jackpot.

To round everyone out, I'll tell you a little about my brother. He's just two years younger than I am, and his birthday is the day after mine. Mom says she held him in, so we could have two separate days. So technically there is an hour between us and two years. Growing up, we looked like twins. Mom always put us in these matching outfits. I was a rather bossy kid; yes, I know it's hard to imagine, and I sure did boss poor Steven around. But we loved each other so much. We did everything together. He was kind of my sidekick. If there was something I wasn't too sure of, I told Steven to try it first, including a cute little furry rat we found, which preceded to bite him. Poor steven had to have a series of rabies shots that even his little cowboy outfit that he was wearing couldn't protect him from. I was in big trouble for that one. Today, I consider him to be one of my best friends as I do my sister. The two of them are very good siblings to have on your side in a bar fight so to speak. In fact, my brother has an impressive tattoo already to flex his muscles on my behalf. Yep, that's right my brother got a big pink breast cancer tattoo on his arm in honor of me. God bless him. One thing my brother said that broke my heart though was when I was first diagnosed, he wished that if anyone had to get sick, he thought it should have been either himself or my sister instead of me. Well, you listen to me, Brother, I did get sick, and I am managing ok. I would never wish for you or Jill to have to go through what I am experiencing. You are an amazing brother and worthy of a full life with happiness and joy. Please go out there and grab your piece of it. It's time for you to have some fun. I need you to let yourself be happy. You are the most amazing brother; please let the world know who you are. Let them see you.

Here and there we have heard some stories about my husband. When I look back, I realize how scary this must have been for him. He is seventeen years older than me, and he thought he was marrying this young chick only to have her die on him leaving him to raise two young children by himself—pretty scary stuff. He never voiced any of that to me. But, you see, his whole life was turned upside down just as much as mine was, or more. I did everything for him. I ran his dental practice; I ran our home; took care of the children; and their personal needs; their education; all the grocery; all the cooking you get the picture here. The man was left in the middle of a lake, in a boat without an oar. I was his oar. Yet, no one really paid too much attention to him or asked him what he needed, or how they could help him; it was all about me. That's a hard place for me to look at, Folks. Yet at the beginning, when I was first diagnosed, he came up with this crazy but cute idea all on his own to have a wig party for me because I was concerned about losing my hair. He invited a bunch of my close friends over for an afternoon, and they all came wearing different types of wigs—some really funny, with multiple colors some with blond bombshell and some just pretty wigs that weren't their hairstyle. My mom came in a blonde wig; the kids even got involved and were wearing wigs. It was a nice afternoon meant to cheer me up, and it was a lovely gesture. However, I was in tunnel vision by then, so I wasn't all there, but I remember it, and I remember that Jere had put this thing together all on his own. It was very thoughtful.

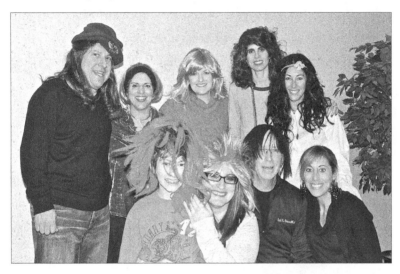

For my birthday the same year he took a whole bunch of my favorite pictures of the family and friends and had them write something, and then he put it all together in this beautiful hardbound book that I still have today. As time goes on, those kinds of things become less but how long do you expect to get all of that all the time. Those were kind and generous things he did during a time when I'm sure he was very scared and unsure of what his life was going to look like. It was nice that he was sort of going through his own tunnel vision, and he just concentrated on getting me well and putting his energy where it could do the most good. And it worked. I thank you for that, Jere. I thank you very much.

I have known Michelle since I was seven years old, and we lived side by side on Walden Road together. She is my family and always will be. As in any long relationship like ours, we have had our ups and downs, but we love each other, and that is a bond that will never break. She is the most beautiful person I know, and when she shines her light on me, everything inside me grows with it. It is her opinion that I cherish the most other than my mother. It is her advice I seek when I am in pain or have a question of judgment. I always have faith in her answers. It is her wonderful parents' condo that has given me respite to write this book alone and in peace. She is the only person that I have allowed to join me at chemotherapy treatments, besides my mother Jere or my sister Jill. That is not a long list, but she is my person. She will always be high on my list. She has that uncanny way of looking at me knowing exactly what I'm thinking or what I may need at any given time. Quite honestly as I am writing this, I am thinking it sounds pretty creepy. Maybe it is, but when you know someone that long, you just don't have to guess any more. You just know. You can just be. You can just rest. That's why I love Michelle.

There are three very close family members that I haven't mentioned yet. We grew up like sisters. I feel as if they are my sisters. If I ever need anything, one or all of them are always there for me. I love them dearly. They are my best of best friends. They are my cousins—my Jodi, Amy, and Liz. Without their unwavering support and their cheerleader approach to my getting better, I'm not sure where I would be today honestly. From each little corner of the world, they live in, they made my life so much better, and they were able to do it from where they were. They are amazing, smart, strong, and beautiful women. Together the four of us really kick some ass. I'm telling you we have a girls' weekend every year and look out when we are in town, cuz we blow it away. Damn! I just adore them and want them to know how much I appreciate everything they do and did for me. I'm so very grateful. They give women a good strong example of women helping women. Jodi, Liz, and I always try to set that same example for our beautiful daughters.

My dad is always there for me. It was tough for him when I got sick as well, especially because he's a little bit more removed from the family. It's difficult for him to join in and get involved in everything. He has been a really good grandfather to my children and has never missed one event of theirs. He has gone to every trick or treat night, every dance recital, piano recital, and everything in between. He gave us our love of the beach, and we enjoy it with him every summer. He likes my cooking, and that makes me giggle. So I cook for him as often as I can. He appreciates it so much; it's really quite cute and complimentary. When we didn't think we were going to be able to get coverage for my radiation treatment, he was right there offering to chip in for the costs. When we finally did go to Indiana for the treatment, he drove a car all the whole ten hours there, just so we would have an extra car and therefore had to fly home by himself. He's like a silent hero sometimes. I don't think people realize how many nice things he does. He takes good care of us and worries about us. When I got sick, he put aside a lot of his personal differences for my behalf, and the whole family now gets together often because he was able to do that. I really appreciated that he was able to do that. It was at great cost to him, and I want to say Thank You, Dad, I love you.

There are so many other family members that were amazing to me—too many to count. I will say to my Uncle Tom and Aunt Sherry, I know you are worried. My Uncle Tom is also my godfather, so I feel a bit closer to him than most I suppose. And boy are he and I a lot alike. He takes good care of my mom and his sister, and I love him for that. I just wanted to tell them I love them, too, and appreciate them always.

I can't complete this chapter without making one more Thank You and telling you a little story. Did I mention that when I started this book, I didn't realize I had never looked back? Now I know I have mentioned it, but I'm not sure I fully explained what that means. When I sat down to begin my story, I had to really concentrate and think hmmm ok what happened?? I had to think really hard. That was a bit confusing. What the hell, it's my story, my life. What's so hard to figure out? It started coming back in flashes, piece by piece, and I was a bucket of tears. It was then that I realized how deep my tunnel vision had been. I had almost put myself into some kind of walking trance of sorts to get myself through this horrible situation while still going through the motions of life. I'm sure people will either want to put me in the loony bin or study me for science once they read this but believe me I was the biggest critic.

Regardless, this is what I believe happened. As the pieces of my journey are coming painfully back to me, so are those of my loved ones that walked a different journey beside me. I explain this to you, so you understand this is how I came to remember a promise that I had made. I promised God that if I could raise my children, that I would help women. Since this chapter is all about Thanking People. I must Thank God for allowing me to raise my children. It has been my greatest gift ever given to me. I have cherished it. It has been my honor to have raised those amazing children. I have loved being a mother, and it has given me great joy. Nothing I have ever done before or will do after will ever compare to being a mother. Now, God, I will keep my promise to you. I thank you for my gift.

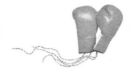

Coping Mechanisms

While writing this book and remembering everything I did to "survive" along the way, I realized just how much I really supported myself. I was there for me when I needed me the most. Now I realize that sounds kooky, and you are probably wondering about my sanity as was I, but I assure you I am mostly sane, so why not wait and hear me out. I just hope I can express myself well enough for you to understand all that I did and all that I accomplished by doing it without realizing it at the time. It is only now when studying it in reverse, do I see some huge obstacles that I was able to accomplish to help myself or to improve my circumstances.

First and foremost, you hear me talking about "Tunnel Vision" all the time. Do you have any idea the strength and fortitude it took for me to put my body and soul into that kind of battle mode, yet still carry out my daily duties? It was as if I was in two places at once. They teach things like that in some Japanese warrior cultures. Where did I come up with that within weeks? How did I accomplish that for such a long period of time? I can't even answer that question, but it is something that is certainly worth analyzing. To be able to compartmentalize on such a monumental scale takes a lot of energy and fierce perseverance. It demonstrates just how dedicated I was to getting well. If I am the only one today with this particular form of aggressive cancer, you can't fault anyone for not making it. This was not an easy thing to accomplish.

I may not have always understood why I was doing what I did to help me survive, but I always understood my motivation. Let me tell you how I—someone who'd never meditated or even read an article on meditation—stumbled upon my own technique. Then let's explore my meditation technique. Here's another interesting story for you all…. When I was first diagnosed, all the doctors kept giving me bottles and bottles of narcotics. This was before the big stink about them, but it didn't mean I didn't understand what they did to you.

Doctor after doctor would prescribe me bottles of these pills with hundreds of them in there. When I questioned one of the physicians, "Why do I need all of these? I'm not really in that much pain".

The response horrified me. He said, "What does it matter? You are terminal anyway; you might as well take them."

I said, "Because I am still a mom, and there is homework to be done and baths to be given and so forth."

He just looked at me, shrugged his shoulders and said, "Suit yourself."

It was at that moment that I was so turned off by pain killers that I don't think in the twenty surgeries I've had to date, I have even gotten through one small prescription. Given that, I had to figure out a way to deal with the pain. Some of it was excruciating. Through it all, somehow my made-up meditation was born. It's actually quite clever, and I am proud to say when my mom was in great pain from a couple surgeries she had, it helped her. It's not really any different than regular meditation, but I had never meditated before, so I didn't know that. It's all in the breathing and controlling it. The greater the pain, the harder you try to control your breath and escape along with it. Just take yourself away little by little with each breath. One time the pain was so severe, I don't remember what was happening, but I do remember being over my body for a short time looking down at the procedure being done to me.

Now, I'm sure that's hard for you all to believe, but it's true. It happened only that one time and never happened again, but I remember it clearly, and, yes, it was very strange. Even though I find myself strange, I don't disagree with my decision to stay away from all those pills. Can you imagine the situation I'd be in today if I had taken all those pills?

As crazy as this sounds, this is also true. Everything I write in this book is my truth. This is what happened to me, and I am trying to give you an honest depiction of what it is like to go through something as horrific as this and still find joy and beauty and love each day I wake. Pause for a second, I must interrupt myself again; bear with me. About eight months prior to being diagnosed with cancer, I was experiencing terrible headaches. Par for the course, I was shuttled from doctor to doctor trying to figure out why I was getting the headaches, and more importantly why and where they were coming from. I had grueling test after test, using me like a lab rat on so many different medications, and they were messing me up big time. I felt like a zombie; I could barely function. I was afraid to get behind the wheel of a car let alone care for my children. Finally, they came up with a diagnosis, Temporal Arteritis—sometimes called Giant Cell Arteritis. Now this is a disease that is in the temporal artery of the brain, and if it's not treated, you could die of a stroke. The strange thing about this is that it is most common among people eighty years old and up. Since I was only half that—forty years old—we were all a bit curious as to how I could have such a problem. Here is the start of why I say I always get everything ten times worse than the average person and twice as complicated. It just is. Needless to say, to prevent a stroke, I was put on high doses of steroids. Most people know that steroids blow you up and can distort your body and make you crazy hungry. That's all true, and I looked like shit, Thank You. But what you may not be aware of is if you are on steroids for an extended period of time, which I was, they alter your brain. In other words, to put it bluntly, they make you PSYCHO!!! I mean you lose control of your temper so easily. You have no patience at all; you just feel out of control. It's an awful feeling. I was in a pickle. I had these two little munchkins to care for that didn't know or understand any of this, and if anything could get under your skin more, it would be them not listening and so on.

Here's where my other little miracle comes in because it took some time and breathing, but I taught myself to even my emotions around them and not fly off the handle. I was kind and patient and loving, and it took every ounce of energy in my body to do that. It was like superhuman strength to keep myself from lashing out at my children. I am most proud of that one. Even though it's not as tangible as the other, I am still most proud of that. When it became intolerable that I couldn't exercise at all for such long periods of time, I negotiated with my doctors. I had always been so active; it was difficult to be trapped in a body that was restricted from anything active. Now again, this is something I may have touched on earlier in the book, but I wanted to tell you how all of this was born.

Because I had developed sarcoidosis of the lung due to my chemotherapy (at least that was the decision at the time), and the treatment for that was steroids. I had just gotten off the steroids after being on them for almost three years, and you know my feelings regarding those nasty little motherfuckers. There wasn't a chance in hell I was going to allow myself to be put back on those. The alternative was to continue my breathing treatments and don't get my heart rate up too high, so I don't get my breathing out of control. Limited as I was, I still wanted to figure out a way to move; I was going stir crazy. I started to go for walks. I needed to be supervised much like a child. That was fun. But my mom called in the cavalry, and my friends showed up, and each day a different person was always around for me to walk with which was nice because we would chat and catch up on the latest town gossip. But eventually that petered out, and it just wasn't enough. The air got cooler, and I was forced to take my walks to the gym on a treadmill. One day I had my headphones in my ears because who wouldn't want to blast some Motown to cheer a girl up, right? I was plugging away, walking and walking, but how can you just walk when "I Heard It from The Grape Vine" is screaming in your ears? I mean, come on people, you have t start wiggling that tush, and so I did, and then I did it some more. The music was so infectious. How could I not until I was into a full-blown dance on the treadmill right in the middle of the gym? That's right, Folks. When the song changed, and Michael Jackson came on, well, my arms started flailing about, and I was just having a good old-time dancing while the treadmill was propelling me into a full-blown, low-impact cardio workout. What do you know? That's how Viki's Crazy Exercise was born. After I realized how many people this could help, I made a video demonstration and am selling it on my website for those that are interested in iamtheone.com. Anyway, what I discovered was this is a lot more than exercise. At one point I started to cry, huge tears of joy running down my face. It became such an outlet for me—not only a way for me to move and get my body in shape but my mind and soul as well. You would be so surprised what it does for you to fully let yourself go without shame or care of who is watching. It's such an uninhibited feeling as no other I had felt before. But it only works if you truly let yourself go. Give yourself up to whatever it is you need at that moment and be able to tune everything out around you and not feel care or embarrassment for the stares and looks you may receive. Because let me tell you, you will get stares and looks. There are headphones in your ears; the people around you cannot hear the beat that you are hearing, not that it would matter to them, but you need to tune that out, not to care about that, to truly let go, and to let your freak flag fly. That's why I call it Viki's crazy exercise. The funny thing is in the end people will surprise you. The only people that came up to me said, "Wow, you look like you are having so much fun up there. I wish my workout was as much fun as yours". I couldn't believe it. I almost fell off the treadmill. We always think the very worst, but it's never usually what it seems, remember that. Don't let things hold you back because you're embarrassed or afraid of what people might think. First of all, we earned the right to live in peace and fly our own kite. Second of all, give people the benefit of the doubt. They aren't always thinking what you conjure up in your head.

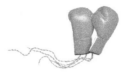

The Big Surgery

All the waiting and healing and discussions with Dr. M. were finally over, and today was the Big Day, my Surgery Day. Oh my, I was a bit nervous; I mean the radical mastectomy was a very long and complicated surgery as we know. I have had many surgeries since, but this was also going to be arduous involving all different areas of my body, so I was going to be hurting pretty good for a while. However, this is something I have agreed to, and not out of only necessity so it's a bit different. As I look up, I see Dr. M. entering into the surgical room where I am doing the prep stuff before surgery; she proceeds to drop a bomb on me. She explains that she found a hernia wrapped around my belly button on the x-ray, and not only will this add to her surgery time (remember I can only be out for so long), but it also complicates things. For me, it takes on a very personal meaning. You see, I had a radical mastectomy, which means, I don't have any nipples. Remember when I referred to myself as a eunuch? Well, that was why. If I have no nipples, and now she's telling me I will have no belly button, I won't have any map. It was too much for me to take in. I needed a point of reference—anything. My body will look like a big white blob with two misshapen mounds on it. I just pleaded with her not to allow this to happen. Dr. M. being the kind of doctor that she is agreed to build me a belly button. But, of course, that was going to take more time. I understood.

Since my memory has returned, and I remember all that we all have been through, walking in the shoes of those I love is .... very difficult. My poor mother and husband waited for thirteen hours. Yes, you heard correctly; that's thirteen hours until Dr. M. came out of surgery. She couldn't keep me under any longer. She had a lot more to do, but she got all the basics done. I had two boobs and a belly button, and I was all closed up. She's freaking amazing. I don't know of anything I could do for thirteen straight hours, do you? Unbelievable!! Even at a nine to five job you mostly sit down, chit chat, go to the bathroom, and have lunch, and that's only eight hours. This surgery was thirteen hours where she was present the entire time doing a very complicated procedure that she ran out of time doing and will have to go back in and prefect. How amazing is that.

I recuperated for quite a while in the hospital after this procedure, and, of course, I got nauseous—always sometime around the second or third day. It's all the anesthesia that gets me backed up which in turn is what brings on the nausea. I can deal with pain better than nausea. I hate being nauseous. UGH!

In addition to my rough hospital stay, I needed lots of physical therapy after this procedure and had to walk with a walker. I think it was a month before I stood fully upright. But I didn't have to wear those horrible itchy painful prosthetics anymore. My goodness, I think I still have scars on my body just from the prosthetics rubbing. The problem is you can only use viable tissue which was why they were trying so hard to expand my tissue, but it just didn't work well.

I kept ending up in the hospital with infections.

They take your tummy and use as much of that as possible, which I didn't have too much of. Now if they went for ass fat, I could not only have great boobs but could probably be a doner (if that was a thing which it isn't, so don't get all excited, Girls). This is the reason I was so sore; they cut through my muscle and everything, so I was a hurting puppy, and you know I had those damn Fucking drains for goodness knows how long that time. I think I blacked out just having to remember.

So that surgery took place in September of 2013 just to give you a time frame for all of this, and Dell's Bar-Mitzvah was November 2012, so I proceeded to have about another five or so surgeries on my reconstruction for the next several years all while still getting chemotherapy—let's not forget. Guess what I am doing, during all this down time while recovering from one surgery after another? Did you guess? I am keeping my promise to my little girl; that's what I'm doing. That's right. I'm planning my little girl's Bat-Mitzvah. It's her turn now. How about that folks??

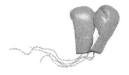

The Bat-Mitzvah

It's Bella's turn, and we know she wants everything her brother got, so it's a challenge to figure out how Mom is going to satisfy that. She wants to be very involved unlike her brother, who could have cared a lick about anything, except to have lots of ice cream and candy. Bella and I really put a lot of thought behind her theme and weekend overall. I'm so proud of her. She is such a cool kid and will grow to be such an amazing person. I'm telling you now, look out for this one, cuz she is going to rule the world one day!

We chose power colors of bright pink and bright orange, very hot, hot, hot, and the theme, of course, was "Girl Power". It was very cool. Isabella came up with all these female singers and vocalists; then she pulled song lyrics from various pieces of work they had done. We then put the name of the artist and lyric on a CD and put them in the middle of the floral arrangement on the kids' tables. She chose a famous female person in history, and we gave the adults all a table with a different famous strong female. On placement cards were the famous quotes that matched each noted woman; you found your table by matching the quote to the woman which was also then at the table. Pretty cool, huh? That kid of mine, she's no shrinking violet. I didn't fight so hard to stay alive, not to take advantage of every moment I had and teach my children what was right and to be strong individuals and that includes especially my daughter.

Now what would one of our parties be like if we didn't do a number? But how could we possibly top the last one? We couldn't, so we go in another direction entirely. Now you need to understand Dell is sixteen at this point, not the eager beaver Isabella was at nine years of age. The fact that we got him out there was something I suppose, but he was clearly not happy about it. Anyway, I digress, back to my idea, since Isabella's hair was such a big focal point of her very being. We got these huge red curly afro-like wigs and put on one-piece bell bottom 70's outfits complete with white patent platform shoes and boots for me. Well, we couldn't have looked more ridiculous. Then we hired the same person who did Dell's dance for us. She did a mashup to Isabella's hip hop dance routine; this time it was complete with her own back-up dancers. We came out to "Dancin' in the Streets" playing imaginary instruments and all, except we flubbed this one up bad and forgot half the steps. I was out there by myself because the girl forgot to cue Jere. It was a huge mess, but no one noticed because we looked so ridiculous, they couldn't stop laughing. Of course, we made sure there was a piano there, and the kids played together for everyone. It was a sight to see—both of my children older now sitting on a piano bench next to one another playing a duet together that they had learned when they tried out and made it for a Piano Extravaganza on a stage with eighteen pianos playing on one stage simultaneously with a conductor. Boy, am I lucky to have such wonderful children. Look at them go. Everyone out of my fog as I watched them come around the bench and take a bow.

This Bat-Mitzvah was no different from the last. It was a weekend celebration. Everyone had come in from out of town again. Some of the people we hadn't seen since Dell's Bar-Mitzvah, so it was lovely to see everyone, and everyone, of course, was happy to see I was still alive and that I didn't make that promise to my daughter in vain—as if I would do such a thing. She was beautiful on the bimah and spoke well. She especially looked lovely the whole weekend in all her outfits. Now did we go shopping or what? Wahoo, did we make a good time of that or what? She's my girl, alright. We took "Grandy" with us for this trip (Grandy is what the kids call my mom— their grandmother), and Grandy didn't disappoint. She sprung for most of the outfits. Where do you think I got my love of shopping from, after all? No, I didn't misspeak—yes outfits plural. You see there are many changes for a young lady during a weekend in her honor after all. I'm not sure which look I favored. She looked so cute in everything, but her party dress was really smashing. We got her a glittery pair of converse sneakers dyed and painted to match. She looked like The Little Mermaid.

We hired the same DJ we had hired for Dell, so he knew us well by then and was having a great time with the kids and adults as well. Again, Isabella's friends were upset. She chose her brother for all the party games, but she knew what she was doing, and the two of them cleaned up! The cousins were older but just as crazy and were dancing and having a ball all over the place. I hope they all share half the joy their parents and I have shared with each other over the years. I would move mountains for them.

I got up and said my speech to Isabella using her hair as an analogy of how it protects her from harm. My lioness daughter uses her hair to hide behind when she doesn't want to face something or is sad, but it flies behind her high and proud when she's happy and free running and beating all the boys in the process. We went back to the house that night for the more intimate party, which is always nice for catching up with those you really wanted to spend more time with and, of course, to change outfits :)

The next morning those that were left straggled in for the bagels and hung for a while until they had to catch their trains, plains, and automobiles. Finally, the house was quiet, except for the four of us sprawled in various places all over the couch half asleep. I thought this scene looked familiar. I'll take it. Eventually, the kids began to squirm. Dell left to take a nap, and Isabella being Isabella went to see if she had any homework due for tomorrow, and off she went. I glanced at Jere; he was out. You know the kind of out that his mouth is open, and an awful noise is coming from his nose and mouth region. I just smiled. I love my family!

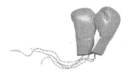

Bucket List

Looks like I made the five-year mark, Holy Shit, How about that? Now, there are just a few things I'd like to do. Call it a Bucket List if you will. I'd like to climb a mountain, and we have been looking, but because of my sarcoidosis of the lung, we are having trouble making that one come true. I'm going to have to settle for a hike or a hill in a foreign land. I want to go ziplining not in the U.S. but through the high trees, where you can see the monkeys and wildlife. I'd like to parasail and ride a ski board in the ocean. I was thinking of jumping out of a plane, but my doctor put the brakes on there and wasn't overly keen on any of this either.

My mom turned seventy-five that January; my sister was to turn fifty-five the upcoming October and me right smack in the center; I was turning fifty. The big 5-0 people, and I was on terra firma. Life couldn't be better. Mom pulled together all her points from her timeshare and her frequent flyer miles and took the three of us on a holiday we would never forget—an all-inclusive trip to Saint Kitts at the Marriott Resort. Boy, it was super nice; the staff was great. We made friends wherever we went. We were having a blast. We even had fun on the plane. It was all inclusive; everything was included: meaning all you could eat and drink. Mom drank some, but Jill and I didn't drink, so we set about checking out the food. We found a fabulous pizza bar and the most amazing cookies you ever tasted. Oh, my goodness, I can smell them now. YUM anyway, then an industrious young cute bartender introduced Jill and I to Rum Punch. OMG, it just tasted like the best Hawaiian punch you ever had. We couldn't believe there was alcohol in these things. Wahoo. Then the party started jumping. That was some good stuff. We were dancing and having ourselves a good ole time.

The next day was the scheduled excursion—my whole reason for being there, not so much Jill's though. Personally, I thought she looked as if she was going to throw up. You see Mom and my sister only reluctantly agreed to take the excursion trip with me and go up to the zipline area. I was so excited but feeling a little bad for them but not really bad— let's be real here. But they sure were good sports. I hired a videographer to mark the moment for us, so we would have the footage to document this for all time. First, they gave us this crazy instructor which was perfect for us. He didn't take too much seriously, and he fit right into our "crazy". We put our equipment on, and it almost weighed as much as me. I tried to go up a hill and fell right back from the weight of the equipment. That happened to me one other time when I backpacked through Europe and over packed my backpack and tried to strap it on from the boot (a boot is the trunk of a car in Europe) and pull it out, and it flung me back in with my legs hanging in the air like a turtle on its back.

After we completed practice, we all hauled ourselves into these big trucks and went up and up and around and up some more and up till we were led off into a dense wooded area and told we needed to hike from here. Well, geez, I guess I got my hike on this one as well. With all the equipment strapped around me and to me, I thought I might collapse, and bear in mind the air was very thin at the altitude level we were at. Finally, I saw Mom and Jill. They looked about like I did.

Then we saw it up in the clouds, yes, you heard that right, in the clouds. The treetops were high; some were below us, but some were close to us; it looked very cool. We walked up a huge platform with a ladder, so we'd have a vantage point to take off from. Our instructor said, "Who wants to go first"; I volunteered loudly; my sister and mother barely said anything. I jumped up through my legs in the air and threw my head back as I was taking off to wave to them. One thing I noticed right away was the quiet and just that beauty of silence. Then I saw the monkeys playing, and that was so beautiful seeing them run free and wild, and that's how I felt for just that moment, free and wild like the monkeys. Then the zipline started flying faster heading on a downhill spiral, and before I knew what was happening, they were capturing me and un-hooking me. As I was righting my sea legs, it was then that I saw Jill coming. She's having a blast for all her worries. If only she could see the joy on her face; she was loving it. Then I blinked, and she was right next to me. Now Mom's going, and we are a bit worried. She's not exactly flailing her arms and singing as Jill and I were, and here she comes, and she hits pretty hard as she comes in. They didn't soften her impact as well as they did with ours. She just sits there a minute. Jill and I are "Are you okay, MOM?"

"Yes, I'm fine, Just give me a second."

The next thing I know, she gets off, and she's dancing the polka around and around with our instructor. That was our awesome zip lining experience, and I wouldn't have wanted to experience it any other way. That was probably the best trip the three of us have ever been on together. There have been others, but there was a magic to this trip that I don't know will ever be outmatched.

That same year Dr. M. said I was finally ready for the HOLY GRAIL. You can just see doves flying if you squint your eyes and a tabernacle choir in the background with their mouths open wide into an OOOOOOO. You can get the picture, I hope. Ok, Ok, I digress ... I get to see the BIG V—no not that Big V; get your heads out of the gutter people, honestly. The big V is the best tattoo guy for areolas. That's all he does. He's known to travel all over the world and do very famous areolas. Just think of all the movie stars that had breast cancer. Let me clarify and say everyone that has a mastectomy doesn't necessarily need areolas. Most nipples can be preserved, and then a tattoo wouldn't be necessary. Unfortunately for me, we know nothing was healthy enough to be preserved, so I've been waiting all these years for enough healing and for most of my surgeries to be complete, so I may get my areolas and complete my map. This is where The Big V comes in. It took me four months to get an appointment; it was worth the wait. I now have my beautiful map. I've got North, South, West, and East. I'm in good shape. I didn't know what to expect when we went there. After all, I'm not exactly what you would call the experienced tattoo girl. I only know of myths that I conjure up in my vast imagination. I was kind of looking forward to letting my bad girl out. Was he going to throw me on the back of his motorcycle and proceed from there? How sterile would the environment be? It was definitely a tattoo parlor, and I had to pay half down four months ago when I made the appointment, but he was here and (very, very tall) and dressed normal—in fact, dressed like an Irish gentleman—very interesting. We went into a private room not out in the middle, where all the others were getting various kinds of tattoos—much as you would expect big dragons and snakes and so forth. There, I was not disappointed, very cool. He covered one side of my chest and asked me a couple of questions like how were they before, and do you like big areolas or small? Should they be dark or light? All kinds of things like that. It was very interesting, and then he began. Jere was so interested he practically had his whole face in there. I'm like, uh, Jere, can you kind of give me a little space?

You're making me feel like a lab rat here. The whole process took about three hours, and they looked fanfuckingtastic. I couldn't believe it. Wow. He gives it a 3D effect, so they really look real even though it's a flat surface. Very cool. I was sore for a while, but shit when haven't I been sore. They still look great today. He said they may fade, and I might want a touch up over time. Okay, I'll let you know when, cuz they still look great.

After the holidays the three stooges (Mom, Jere, and I) decided to use some of Jere and my points and head to the Grand Cayman Islands. None of us had ever been there before, so we thought we'd give it a try, and I could cross off a few of my things on my bucket list. Well, the place was beautiful but very expensive. We all thought we had been to places just as nice that were not half as costly. But it didn't take away from the beauty of the place nor the fun we had. First, we went out on this big boat where you could go parasailing off the boat. We suit up and Jere and I go together. It whisks us off the boat, and you are really freaking high up. It's so gorgeous. You can barely make out the boat. I'm swinging my legs and waving my arms to everyone down there. They are sort of frantically waving up at me and pointing. I don't understand why, so I kind of hang upside down and yell "Helllooo out there. Ahoy Mateys". I thought I was being very funny after all, and then I saw they were pointing next to me, so I looked over and realized that Jere was hanging over the other side vomiting his little heart out. Oh my, I am the world's worst wife. I signal for them to bring us down, and I start cleaning him up trying not to laugh. I go get him some of my nausea medication that I always have on hand and begin to see some color starting to come back into his face. We headed back to our lounge after that and let Jere take his nap with fifteen towels wrapped around him and his head.

He looked like a cross between a mummy and a dork—a dork-mummy. Mom and I moved a couple chairs down from him not only to escape the smell of vomit but the embarrassment as well. Ah poor Jere.

The next couple of days on the trip we took out ski boats and went as fast as we could in the ocean. The funny thing was Mom was the crazy fastest of all of us. I kept getting caught up in the waves but not mom. I would look over at her, and my seventy-eight year old mother would be flying over the waves taking air like a stunt woman, and Jere and I were going fifteen miles an hour barely flopping over the waves. To put it mildly, we were pathetic, and my mother was a Rock Star!! Between the parasailing and ski boats, we decided to stick to what we knew best for the rest of the trip ... shopping. That was an area we had no problem mastering. We ate, sunbathed, and shopped all and all; we had a good time. The three stooges ruled again.

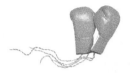

The Marathon

In the Fall of 2016, I was five years hanging in there so to speak, and my family decided to get all involved in the Susan G. Komen Race for the Cure Half Marathon in New York City. Now you must understand the huge undertaking this was for our family. Each person that walked had to raise about two thousand dollars. In addition, there were team T- shirts that had to be made, hotel arrangements, and so and on. It was a huge endeavor. But my awesome family got it in their heads that they wanted to do this in my honor. What do you do with that?? How do you pull a lottery ticket like the one I have? It's priceless. I just didn't know what to do with all the emotion bubbling inside me.

Thinking back on it now, I am trembling with pride for my family. It's funny; they were there to honor me, but it was really all of them that were the stand-out heroes. They just couldn't see how amazing they all were. That's where I got my true strength from. It was them all along. They are all so remarkable.

We had so much fun for months planning just to get to New York. We all had our strengths, so we pulled together and divided and conquered. I was pretty adept at fundraising, so I just kept at it and did as much as I could to cover anyone that didn't meet their goal. We went to the stores that Mom and I walk into every month when I have to walk off my sick, as I call it before I can get back into the car after chemotherapy. Two of our favorite stores had events in my honor and gave the proceeds to me for the marathon. Now how nice was that?? We have walked those lanes and talked to the shop keeps for so many years we have become so friendly with many of them. It was so kind of them to do that for me. In addition, my good friend that owns a boutique store at home in Harrisburg had a fundraiser for me as well. She has always come through for me. She is kind and generous and has the best clothes in Harrisburg. All my clothes come from her. Between all those fundraisers and then Capital Blue and some of my old haunts who gave me money, we were well set. My cousins brought in money as well, so as a family, we rocked it!!

My cousin who lives in New York took care of getting us all the hotel rooms. Boy, was that a job. Poor Jodi, she was never gonna win that one. No one was going to be happy there. Jodi also did the T- shirts. OMG, they rocked. We had the best team T-shirts EVER!!! We were such a cool family.

Meanwhile, there were a huge bunch of all different ages between our group, and everyone was going to walk at different paces and distances. We were trying to keep track of us all and team up. We had my mom and Uncle Tom and Aunt Sherry. They were all not walking too much and going to keep an eye on the children and meet up with us at key areas like the Brooklyn Bridge and fun places like that. Then there was Phyllis who is the mother-in-law of my cousin Amy, but she and I became best friends. This event is where I got to know her best and started calling her my adopted mother-in-law.

The walk is a special place for Phyllis and me. I will remember it as our change in relationship. I think my cousin Liz would feel the same. Liz is a riot; she met up with us while we were breaking for lunch. She was only planning to see us for a bit and was wearing her "cute shoes" which is so Liz. It's what I love about her. But being Liz, she ended up walking the last five miles with us complaining the whole way. Poor Phyllis, had to entertain her with lavish stories to keep her occupied, so she wouldn't concentrate on her aching feet. Phyllis is an excellent storyteller. Liz made it to the finish line. Bless her sweetheart. Then we have my other cousins, Amy, and Jodi, and they came with their husbands Jake and Adam as well as their children— two girls for Jodi and two boys for Amy, but it was just women walking really, so the guys held down the fort with the kids and mom and uncle Tom. Amy and Jodi are very active and put us all to shame. They have legs of steel. To round out our little group was my daughter Isabella—just thirteen but remember she's a tough one—my little lion. Amy and Jodi also found her a very good conversationalist. I say this because I got lost from everyone. But I'll tell you that in a minute. What I didn't say was not only did we have these awesome T-shirts—remember when

I referred to my good friend that has the store in Harrisburg—well, she also got us all these really cool breast cancer tights. We all picked out the ones we wanted in advance of the walk. Arm in arm, we marched down the street with our cool Tee's wearing our fancy tights. We looked like Grease Lightning. (You know, like from the movie when Olivia Newton John had those black painted on tights?

We looked way better) Go Grease Lightning Go!! YAY.

Wherever you looked, there was a sea of pink. It was crazy. I had never participated in anything like this before. People were wearing costumes and tutus. They had their faces painted. It was a very joyful walk. Everyone had a story. People had names written on their shirts. Many were walking for those that they had loved and had passed from this horrible disease. Some walked for those that couldn't walk. Some pushed people in wheelchairs. It really was a moving scene, and in the middle of the sea of pink, I got lost. I needed to sit down and rest, and the next thing I knew everyone was swallowed up by that sea of pink.

I wasn't sure I could walk much more anyway, and it was getting quite cold. I thought possibly I could take one of the shuttles to the finish line and wait for everyone. When I tried to get in one of the shuttles, it turned out the driver was going in another direction. I got out and didn't see another shuttle again for the rest of the day. While I sat and pondered my problem, two women sat down beside me. They were wearing the craziest of outfits. Pink tutus and had their hair in whirly head bands and faces painted, but what was sobering were the names written on their shirts. Being me, I started up a conversation with them. The two were best friends and walking on behalf of a co-worker and the aunt of one of the women—I don't recall which. They were lovely. I told them about my awesome family and me and that I was kind of stuck. We decided to walk together. We didn't think it was that far (boy, were we mistaken). I set off with my new friends to finish the journey. Might as well I thought. Originally, it was never my intention to walk so much. I didn't really think I could do that, and no one else wanted me, too, so that's why no one was really looking for me. They never suspected that I would be stuck and attempting to complete the walk. We did have phones, and I eventually called and let them know I was with these terrific women that were watching out for me, and I was okay. They were all just ahead of us. It was getting quite cold by now and the sun was starting to go down and my legs were quite sore. It was a good thing these women were good conversationalists. I was also starting to get hungry. They had water and food stations all along the route, but now that we were nearing the end, there wasn't anything. However, I did notice a lot of ambulances trolling up and down which wasn't very reassuring to me. I was tempted to call out and say "Hey, give me a ride to the finish", but I'm no quitter!! And I'm certainly no pussy! Onward I went—maybe a bit hunched over but onward. Finally, we rounded a corner, and we saw a line of people clapping and yelling. It was very exhilarating. I had never even run a small race before, so I was amazed at the fan fair and how it made you feel. I kind of felt like a super star as if I had accomplished something amazing considering my condition.

When I got closer to the top, I saw my cute family. Adam and Jake quickly ran to me and gave me one of those silver blankets that keep you very warm. Jake gave me some almonds. Those guys have been watching out for me ever since they married my favorite people in the world. I'm pretty lucky that way. I'll tell ya. Then Mom gives me a huge hug, and Uncle Tom and Aunt Sherry, too. All the kids are running around playing, and it's such a lovely scene. Somehow, I got ahead of Amy and Jodi and everyone because it must have been a good twenty minutes before they rounded the hill looking exhausted but happy. My Bella included; except she didn't look very exhausted. We all hugged. Liz was so funny. Her daughter met us there. Gabby is so sweet and was very proud of mom.

I took stock as I looked at the chaos around me. My whole family is here, but for a few family members, and all these other amazing women who have conquered or are celebrating the lives of others that they have lost to this terrible disease called Breast Cancer, I honor and celebrate them. I realize how very blessed I am. I look at my crazy family all running around in circles freezing and in various forms of pink, exhausted after a very long day but laughing. We were all together, and that's what we celebrate the most. They all came here to celebrate me and my accomplishment, and the fact is it's really about the joy of us all being together—being intact. They are my strength to propel me forward for another five years and more. They are where I draw my energy to move one foot in front of the other each day when I must fight with the insurance companies, or my joints hurt so bad it's difficult to get out of bed. But this amazing family gives me that strength to pull myself up by my bootstraps and get myself out of that bed. They are the sun and the moon and the stars.

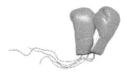

Epilogue

That's my crazy story, Folks. I told you it would be a bit of a roller coaster ride. But you all survived as I will go on to do. I am a very determined woman. I have my promise to God to keep, and I keep my promises. I plan on hanging around because not only do I have a lot more to do, but I'm having far too much fun. Because guess what? "I'm the luckiest girl around. I just happen to have cancer".

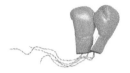

Dedication

I wrote this book out of a desire to tell my story my way. In my own words and a full true accounting of what I did or went through for the love of my children Isabella and Dell. I dedicate this book to them. They are the greatest gifts I have ever been given and raising them has been a privilege and an honor. I loved being a mother more than anything. It's been my most precious gift that I hold in my heart for all my days. I thank you, Dell and Isabella, for allowing me the privilege of being your mom. I hope you'll read this story to your children one day and tell them you were loved very much.

I would like to thank Tyger for coming into my life and bringing a smile and light to my heart. You are a special young man.

Thank You, Kirsten, for all my beautiful clothes. Everyone always asks me where I get them.

You can contact Kirstin at The Plum in Harrisburg at 717-737-8153 or check out her website at www.the-Plum-West theplumclothing.com

Thank You, Jim Muligan, for all my awesome glasses. If you want, you can get in touch with Jim at Bouquet Mulligan DeMaio Eye Professionals, at 717-272-0581, at http://bmdeye.com

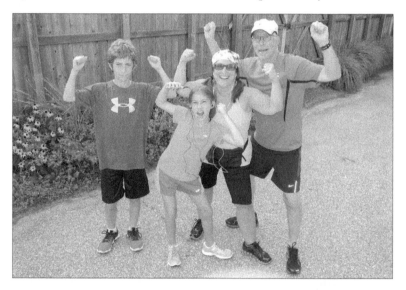